LOCAL HEALTH POLICY IN ACTION

LOCAL HEALTH POLICY IN ACTION

The Municipal Health Services Program

Eli Ginzberg
Edith M. Davis
Miriam Ostow

and Associates:

Patricia Maloney Alt
Albert A. Bocklet
Ann Lennarson Greer
David E. Hayes-Bautista
George Dorian Wendel

LandMark Studies
Rowman & Allanheld
PUBLISHERS

ROWMAN & ALLANHELD

Published in the United States of America in 1985
by Rowman & Allanheld, Publishers
(a division of Littlefield, Adams & Company)
81 Adams Drive, Totowa, New Jersey 07512

Library of Congress Cataloging in Publication Data

Ginzberg, Eli, 1911-
  Local health policy in action.

  (LandMark studies)
  Includes index.
  1. Municipal Health Services Program (U.S.)   2. Com-
munity health services—United States.   3. Urban health—
United States.   I. Davis, Edith M.   II. Ostow, Miriam.
III. Municipal Health Services Program (U.S.)   IV. Title.
[DNLM: 1. Community Health Services—United States.
2. Health—United States.   3. Health Policy—United States.
WA 546 AA1 G4L]
RA445.G54   1985   362.1'0973   84-27524
ISBN 0-8476-7425-8

85 86 87 / 10 9 8 7 6 5 4 3 2 1
Printed in the United States of America

Contents

Tables

Foreword

This brief Foreword has one purpose, to set the book that follows within the context of its subject, the Municipal Health Services Program (MHSP), a project initially designed and funded by the Robert Wood Johnson Foundation and subsequently expanded in scope through the partnership of the Health Care Financing Administration (HCFA) of the Department of Health and Human Services (HHS).

MHSP was a multisite demonstration in the delivery of primary care to urban populations. Five cities, Baltimore, Cincinnati, Milwaukee, St. Louis, and San Jose, were the sites chosen to determine whether, with local mayoralty leadership, ambulatory health care services to the inner-city poor through the establishment and expansion of neighborhood health care centers could be improved. The demonstration commenced in 1978 and was formally terminated (although some funds remained to be spent later) in 1984. The U.S. Conference of Mayors and the American Medical Association participated with the Johnson Foundation as cosponsors of MHSP.

This volume presents the findings and recommendations that were developed by the Conservation of Human Resources, Columbia University as a result of their evaluation of the program for the Johnson Foundation. Principal responsibility for designing and carrying out this evaluation was shared by Mrs. Miriam Ostow, Senior Research Scholar, and myself in collaboration initially with Dr. Michael Millman and later Ms. Edith Davis of the Conservation staff. We were further mutually assisted by our field associates, the importance of whose contribution is indicated by their listing on the title page as coauthors of this work.

It should be emphasized that ours was one of two evaluations that were performed. HCFA made a grant to Professor Ronald Andersen, the Director of the Center for Hospital Administration Studies (CHAS), Graduate School of Business, the University of Chicago, to undertake a study of the utilization, costs, and use of alternative providers found at the demonstration sites and this comparison report is currently nearing publication.

It was agreed from the outset that the focus of our evaluation would be the process by which political, community, professional, and organizational forces alternately facilitated and retarded the transformations in the public system of health care delivery that the program sought to effect.

To provide a firm base for assessing the transformations brought about as a result of the program we prepared an historical baseline volume (Edith Davis and Michael L. Millman, *Health Care for the Urban Poor,* Rowman & Allanheld, 1983) which described the system of ambulatory care in each of the five demonstration cities as of the initiation of the program. For those who want to see the demonstration whole, a review of the earlier volume would prove helpful.

The remainder of the Foreword will outline for the prospective reader the sequencing of the successive chapters and their contents. Chapter 1 provides an overview of the program that was initiated in each of the five cities with information as to how services were delivered and utilized.

Chapter 2 focuses on resources, outlines the revenues used to cover the program costs including the Medicare and Medicaid waivers that were made possible through the collaboration of HCFA together with assistance from several of the states in the case of the Medicaid waivers.

In Chapter 3 attention is directed to changes in the national health care environment during the course of the demonstration, especially the tightening of the money spigots and the impact on the development and the shape and scope of the program.

Chapter 4 is the "meat" of the evaluation, in the sense that it traces out the ways in which the behavior of the different interest groups- political, health professional, and community—intersected with the goals of the program and facilitated or retarded their accomplishment.

Chapter 5 provides a summary which highlights the more important lessons and implications which we were able to infer from our five-year evaluation effort.

Chapter 6, the last, views the program and the evaluation in a larger context. The chapter asks and seeks to answer the question: What is the potential of community health care centers to improve the quantity and quality of health care for low-income individuals and families living in the inner-city? Not to give our conclusions away, let me say that we anticipate both potential and limitations for these centers in the cost constraining environment that lies ahead.

Prior to the initiation of the MHSP, Conservation of Human Resources, in its almost forty years of continuous operation, had never engaged in evaluative studies. Its primary focus has been policy research. There was some reluctance, therefore, on our part to undertake the MHSP evaluation. However, I am pleased to report that it proved to be a challenging effort from which we have gained new and deeper insights into the complex ways in which government, providers, and the public must interact if patients are to receive a reasonable quantity and quality of the services they need to function effectively at an affordable price.

We hope that the reader of the present volume will find enough information to determine what makes a difference in the ongoing search for ways to improve health care services for the low-income urban population. That is our aim and aspiration.

Eli Ginzberg, Director
Conservation of Human Resources
May 1985

Research Staff

Conservation of Human Resources, *Columbia University*:

Eli Ginzberg, Director
Miriam Ostow
Edith M. Davis (1980–1984)
Charles Brecher
Michael L. Millman (1977–1980)
Maury Forman (1977–1983)
Penny Peace

Field Associates:

Baltimore:
Patricia Maloney Alt, *University of Baltimore*

Cincinnati:
Albert A. Bocklet, *Xavier University*

Milwaukee:
Ann Lennarson Greer, *University of Wisconsin-Milwaukee*

St. Louis:
George Dorian Wendel, *Saint Louis University*

San Jose:
David E. Hayes-Bautista, *University of California-Berkeley*

Acknowledgments

In the preparation of this volume, which is a reconstruction of the course of the Municipal Health Services Program (MHSP) and an assessment of its achievements, the authors benefitted from the ongoing assistance of several groups of colleagues. Their generosity is all the more noteworthy since many of them had also contributed to our earlier baseline volume, *Health Care for the Urban Poor* (Edith Davis and Michael L. Millman, Rowman & Allanheld, 1983).

Our colleagues Dr. Ronald Andersen and Dr. Gretchen Fleming of the Center for Health Services Administration (CHAS) at the University of Chicago, who conducted a parallel evaluation of the program in terms of its utilization, costs, and influence upon patient care-seeking behavior, willingly shared their data and perceptions with us and these helped to illuminate our findings reached through a different research methodology. Dr. Tony Hausner, project officer at HCFA which sponsored the CHAS research, coordinated our activities and made available data derived from the Medicare and Medicaid waiver program.

Dr. Carl Schramm, Andrew Green, and Gary Christopherson, who collaborated in the central administration of the MHSP, provided us with program management reports and insights into the dynamics of program implementation from the purview of external management.

The partnership of our field staff in the evaluation is evident from the title page. Less apparent, however, is the indispensable assistance of their research assistants who performed much of the tedious raw data collection and processing. The inputs of the many public officials and their staffs as well as those of the local program management in each of the sites, while invisible, must not go unrecognized. We are indebted to each and all of them for what we succeeded in learning of the daily life of the MHSP.

Finally, the preparation of the manuscript for publication was made possible by the technical skills, the cooperation, the patience, and the good humor of the support staff at Conservation, notably Ellen Levine and Shoshana Vasheetz, and the administrative assistance of Charles Frederick.

1

Introduction
The Demonstration and Its Setting

In the mid-1970s the Robert Wood Johnson Foundation began to explore
the feasibility of launching a significant demonstration of public,
community-based service delivery to inner-city residents. The effort would
be a logical next-step in its program commitment to the expansion of
access to primary care. The many difficulties that confronted such an
undertaking were evident: the receding ability and interest of local
government to address the service problems of the poor and the indigent
after a decade or more of aggressive federal leadership; the powerlessness
of the popular constituency and a corresponding lack of responsiveness on
the part of local political leadership; the political problems that new,
sponsored health care programs might evoke by competing with the few
private physicians who continued to practice in low-income neighborhoods; the bureaucratic isolation of health departments from local municipal hospitals that would hinder, if not block, the goal of shifting patients
from hospital emergency rooms to neighborhood clinics; and the
difficulties of stretching and supplementing current revenues to cover what
was intended to be a substantial increase in both the quantity and quality
of care to be rendered.

In reaching an affirmative decision to appropriate $15 million for a
five-year, five-city demonstration program despite so substantial a risk factor, the Johnson Foundation was influenced by the willingness of two
prominent organizations—the U.S. Conference of Mayors and the American Medical Association—to cosponsor the effort.

In addition to explicitly confirming the importance of the project, this
collaboration offered support in two critical arenas. First, an assurance by

the Conference of Mayors of the active interest and participation of the chief elected official in each of the cities materially enhanced the likelihood of success. And second, the involvement of the American Medical Association could help garner the support of local physicians and avoid or at least moderate concerns and conflicts over the issue of competition with private practice.

In 1977 the Foundation appointed an advisory committee, under the chairmanship of Dr. Robert Ebert, president of the Milbank Memorial Fund and former dean of the Harvard Medical School, whose membership included representatives of the cosponsoring organizations as well as of the larger medical community and the public.

The first and principal task of the advisory committee was to formulate the selection criteria and to designate the sites to receive awards. It was decided to invite proposals from the nation's 50 largest cities and then to identify, on the basis of the formal submissions and site visits by the advisory committee and the Foundation staff, those that showed the best promise of a rapid buildup of quality ambulatory services at a network of at least three comprehensive health care centers in the inner city.

The proposals were judged by their potential for realizing the primary goal of the demonstration, to broaden access to ambulatory care for low-income inner-city residents through local government action to restructure the public health care delivery system. This goal was objectified in a set of interrelated programmatic efforts that included shifting the locus of care from the emergency room and the outpatient clinics of the public hospital to neighborhood health centers; integrating traditional preventive care with therapeutic services; and offering comprehensive services to all members of the community, without distinctions of age, sex, or clinical category.

Recognizing the long-term fiscal constraints of local government, the Foundation stipulated there should be no incremental commitment of resources to the program; rather, it anticipated a shift in funding and personnel from the public hospital to the neighborhood health clinic to parallel the projected shift in patients and the concomitant reduction in the scale of hospital operations.

Another goal of the program was to improve the continuity of care by enabling physicians who staffed the centers to follow their patients upon hospitalization. In addition, it was thought that the expansion of neighborhood health centers would present an opportunity to experiment with new forms of service delivery through the utilization of a large complement of mid-level providers, particularly nurse practitioners and physician assistants.

The program also looked forward to the enrollment within the centers of a broad segment of the population, not only the poor and indigent but also insured persons capable of paying for their care. If that objective were achieved, it would augur well for the viability of the centers once the Foundation grant came to an end.

The Foundation recognized from the outset that the accomplishment of these many difficult and diverse goals, involving multiple sectors of municipal and county government, would require the continuing commitment and leadership of a senior elected official, whom the Municipal Health Services Program (MHSP) design identified as the mayor.

In developing the program the advisory committee enlisted an important collaborator whose contribution—direct and indirect—of financial resources to the demonstration exceeded by a considerable amount the total sum of philanthropic dollars committed by the Foundation. That collaborator was the Health Care Financing Administration (HCFA) of the U.S. Department of Health and Human Services (HHS). The Foundation staff, headed by Dr. Robert Blendon, succeeded in gaining the support of senior officials of HCFA to enter into a partnership under which the MHSP sites became eligible for both Medicare and Medicaid waivers that provided additional sources of funding for an expanded service program. The waivers offered two principal benefits to enrollees: they enabled the sites to provide services to the elderly and the poor without the mandatory deductible and copayments; and they permitted the sites to offer additional services, both therapeutic and preventive, of which the most important proved to be dentistry, eye care, podiatry, and immunization. Perhaps the chief advantage to the centers was the ability to be reimbursed at an institutional rate, comparable to a hospital outpatient department, rather than at fee-for-service rates paid to individual practitioners.

A major by-product of the partnership with HCFA was the development of a large-scale evaluation effort to determine the effect of the demonstration on the quantity and quality of the health care services obtained by the inner-city populations participating in the program, as well as its effect on costs of care in comparison to a control group of patients utilizing alternative sources of care (both private practitioners and hospital emergency rooms and clinics). HCFA entered into a contract with the Center for Health Administration Studies (CHAS), University of Chicago, and its director, Professor Ronald Andersen, to perform this evaluation.

In accordance with its established practice, the Foundation provided for a concurrent evaluation of the program to be undertaken by the Conservation of Human Resources (CHR), Columbia University, Professor Eli Ginzberg, director. This effort was designed to monitor the process of change in each city and to assess the elements that facilitated or impeded the structural alterations specified in the proposal. The legislative, bureaucratic, professional, and community organizational dimensions of the project were the foci for data gathering and analysis.

Announcement of the program in 1977 and initial solicitation of proposals from among the nation's 50 largest cities elicited 41 inquiries followed by the submission of formal proposals from 28 cities. The final selection was made in May 1978 and the award-winning cities—Baltimore, Cincinnati, Milwaukee, St. Louis, and San Jose—publicly announced in June 1978.

As is true for most selective procedures, there were differences of opinion as to the criteria that should receive special weight in the final ranking, from the strength of the public health care delivery system in place to the feasibility of the designs developed to reform and improve the extant system. The fact that the MHSP was conceived as a national demonstration and its sponsors were national organizations—the Robert Wood Johnson Foundation, the U.S. Conference of Mayors, the American Medical Association, and ultimately the federal government—implied that the selection committee would seek to achieve a reasonable geographic representation (no more than one site in any state), and to include at least one city with a large Hispanic presence so that the target population would not be exclusively urban blacks. As is apparent, the final selection was sensitive to both considerations.

An important element in the design of the program was the recognition by the Foundation of the need for a strong management unit that would have continuing oversight of the progress of the grantee cities in implementing their proposals within a reasonable time frame. Implementation involved a number of complex steps, starting with the appointment of a citywide project director and individual site managers; site selection; the purchase of property and construction in the case of new health centers; facility conversion/expansion of existing centers; and staffing of each of the sites. Actions to stimulate enrollment and to expand utilization as rapidly as possible; establishment of financial controls and billing/collection systems; and the development of operating procedures for new centers as well as modification of existing procedures in older centers that were integrated into the demonstration, were all necessary implementation measures.

The central administration of the MHSP, initially based at the New York Hospital-Cornell Medical Center under the direction of Richard Berman, was moved to Johns Hopkins University when Berman resigned to become chief of the Office of Health Systems Management of New York State. He was followed first by Charles Buck, then by Carl Schramm who remained at the helm from 1980 until the termination of the program. Two successive assistant directors carried much of the day-to-day responsibility, Andrew Greene and Gary Christopherson.

The effective authority of the central administration of MHSP was reinforced by the stipulation of the Foundation that the quarterly release of grant funds to the participating cities would be conditioned upon their meeting specified performance goals for the preceding quarter. This meant that the Foundation kept a tight rein on the release of its money and the mayor and mayoral staff were under continuing pressure to adhere to agreed-upon schedules for opening and operating the clinics, expanding their utilization, and meeting stipulated criteria of staffing, costs, scope of services, and other operational goals.

The central administration did much more, however, than hold local officials to performance standards, important as that task was throughout the course of the demonstration. It also served as informal consultant to the local project managers who sought advice and assistance in technical as well as political areas. When conflicts erupted among community groups or bureaucratic resistances threatened the progress of the demonstration, the management group was able to intervene and perform a critical negotiating role. On the few occasions when a local program confronted a major personnel or financial difficulty, the management team once again was able to interject itself and work out constructive resolutions. Control over the timely distribution of the grant monies provided the management team with the crucial tool needed to prod, guide, advise, check, criticize, encourage, and otherwise assist each of the cities to proceed close to schedule in the highly complex effort of improving the system of ambulatory health care for its target population.

The complexity of the demonstration has been suggested by the multiple sources of funding for its operations (the Foundation, HCFA, local and state governments [Medicaid waivers], private insurance, and self-pay); the three sponsoring organizations (the Foundation, the U.S. Conference of Mayors, and the American Medical Association); its pyramidal administrative structure topped by the central management team based at Johns Hopkins; and the two evaluation efforts, based respectively at Columbia University and at the University of Chicago.

Achievement of its principal goal, the reorganization of the public system of ambulatory care, of necessity engaged the interest, if not the participation, of a broad range of parties. Within each city, responsibility was shared, at a minimum, by two major bureaucracies, the department of health and the municipal hospital, whose members had widely different goals and competences and seldom interacted with each other. Governance was still another major variable. Some cities were governed by strong mayors and in others the mayor shared much of the decision-making power with other local officials. In three of the five cities, the public hospital was not under the jurisdiction of the mayor but was controlled and operated by the county or the state.

The role of neighborhood-based groups, which was integral to the design of the program, varied noticeably. In some cities they were highly organized and exercised their political clout to influence the location of new clinics and the selection of existent sites for expansion. In other cities they had relatively little initial leverage on shaping the program.

Another variation in the design and implementation of the demonstration derived from the role of the medical school; in some cases it was closely affiliated with the referral hospital(s) that served the MHSP clinic patients and in others it had only a remote responsibility for the inpatient and specialty needs of these patients.

Many other elements, such as voluntary hospitals, physician groups, and overarching local political issues could be identified, which were important influences in some of the demonstrations and relatively silent in others. Variability aside, though, in each demonstration the array of forces in the political, bureaucratic, professional, and community environments that influenced the established patterns of delivery of ambulatory health care to the inner-city population were large and diverse; and the demonstration that was aimed at expanding and improving the delivery of such services, at an affordable cost, could succeed, even modestly, only through a realignment and an accommodation of the goals of these competing, often conflicting, interest groups.

The evaluation of the implementation of the MHSP, whose findings form the substance of this volume, was a similarly complex undertaking. As noted earlier, this evaluation, performed by the Conservation of Human Resources (CHR), Columbia University, limited its function to monitoring and assessing the process of change and the resistances to change in the political-institutional environment that bounded the demonstration. Outcome evaluation, in terms of the critical measures of utilization and cost of the program, was the focus of the University of Chicago effort. The methodology adopted by the CHR evaluation assumed that the gathering and preliminary analysis of data on the political-institutional dimensions of the program could be performed most reliably by an astute participant observer, who could follow the day-by-day vicissitudes of the demonstration from the vantage of his familiarity with the local environment. This methodology was developed by Dr. Richard Nathan, formerly of the Brookings Institution and now at Princeton University, a pioneer in the field of evaluation research. Originally applied to the study of major federal programs, including Public Service Employment (PSE), it was adapted by CHR to the MHSP effort.

It essentially monitors the process of program implementation utilizing a variety of nonquantitative techniques and data sources such as document analysis, media review, interviewing, close observation of official action (legislative, executive, and judicial) and responses by the community and the private and voluntary sectors. These analyses extend and serve to interpret the conventional operations and outcome data as a means of evaluating program success or failure and the contributing factors and causes. To assure comparability of findings and conclusions from site to site in the case of national or area/regional programs, uniform reporting protocols are developed to guide the locally-based observers. These reports are then analyzed and synthesized by a central staff which is responsible for formulating conclusions about the total program experience and its implications for future policy and programmatic action.

For its evaluation of the MHSP, the CHR staff received quarterly reports from each of the field associates. These reports were supplemented by periodic visits to consult each of the associates on his or her own territory, and an annual conference of the field associates as a group in New York City together with the director, the senior research associate, and the MHSP evaluation project manager to review developments over the past 12 months and to chart new directions for the coming year. The opportunity for an intensive interchange between the field associates and the CHR staff as well as with each other proved a source of additional insight. The field associates also participated in the annual meetings of the MHSP advisory board to review the progress of the demonstration, which were attended by representatives of the Foundation, project and site managers, government officials, and the staffs of both evaluation projects.

It must be obvious that the success of this methodology depended heavily for its nonquantitative data upon the access of the field associate to the numerous individuals involved in the administration, planning, operation, and oversight of the project in his city, their cooperation and their candor. The task was facilitated by the Foundation, which conditioned its funding of each proposal upon an agreement to participate in both evaluation projects in addition to furnishing regular operating and financial reports to the treasurer and the central administration staff.

What the Foundation could not dictate, however, was the motivation of diverse individuals and groups concerned with the demonstration to apprise the field associates of critical developments and to offer their interpretations, explanations, and assessments of events. Given the continuing pressures of the program there was little incentive and conceivably a disincentive to furnishing information to the field associate. Intimacy with behind-the-scene details of local program implementation might result in disclosures to the management team at Johns Hopkins or to the Foundation at Princeton that would adversely affect the project's future requests for financial or other assistance. To counteract these concerns, CHR provided public assurance that information obtained locally for the evaluation effort would not be shared either with the central team or the Foundation.

The question of confidentiality was, however, only one prong of a two-pronged issue. The other stemmed from the virtual lack of feedback and any practical assistance to the local project and site managers that was a necessary consequence of the uncompromising neutrality of the evaluation. CHR avoided the role of consultant to optimize project operations. Its arm's-length stance extended to the local administrative team as well as to the central and Foundation staffs. Therefore, local managers had little to gain, even as they recognized that they did not run any risks from responding openly to the field associates. Reciprocity would have been a preferred basis for their interaction with the evaluation.

So much for the structuring of the demonstration and for the CHR evaluation. What about the setting in which the demonstration was carried out? In 1983, CHR published *Health Care for the Urban Poor* (Edith M. Davis and Michael L. Millman, Rowman & Allanheld, Totowa, N.J.), its initial report of MHSP, which reconstructed in considerable detail the changing environment for health care delivery in the five cities from the period of the Great Society of President Johnson to the New Federalism of President Reagan. Since this baseline report is available, we need call attention here only to the more important changes that occurred in the interval between the origins of the MHSP and the termination of the five-year demonstration period in late 1983.

The feasibility of undertaking a project of the nature and scale of the MHSP was under exploration at the time when President Carter entered the White House, that is, early in 1977. It is necessary to recall that Medicare and Medicaid had then been in operation for a decade; that the Congress (and state legislatures) were becoming increasingly concerned about accelerating health care costs; that the winning candidate for the presidency had run on a platform endorsing early action to establish national health insurance; that the nation was just emerging from a recession which had driven the employment rate to 9 percent, its highest level since World War II; that the American public still favored the elaboration of social welfare benefits. The expansion of health care, in particular, continued to attract widespread public support.

Within this generally expansionary climate, the health policy community delineated a number of priority issues. Access to health care was still impeded by the tautness in the supply of physicians, particularly physicians able and willing to practice among the rural and urban poor. Each year saw general practitioners in low-income areas retire or die with no successors to replace them. As a consequence, more and more of the urban poor had no alternative but to seek care from the emergency rooms and outpatient departments of hospitals located in or close to the community where they lived.

But this alternative was also seriously constrained. In many cities, voluntary hospitals that served impoverished neighborhoods could no longer balance their books and accordingly relocated, merged, or closed their doors. At the same time, local public hospitals were facing major hurdles of deteriorating plant, difficulties in maintaining adequate staff, and a shortage of tax revenues to cover those who sought free care.

In 1976 a national commission was established to study the future of public general hospitals under the sponsorship of the Hospital Research and Educational Trust and the chairmanship of Arthur Hess. Nationwide, there was growing uncertainty about the role of the public hospital in a system dominated by private insurance and public financing programs such as Medicare and Medicaid which entitled their beneficiaries to free choice of provider with the resultant shift of a considerable portion of the public hospital's patients to the private sector.

Concomitant with ever larger federal outlays for social welfare programs, there was a steady erosion of municipal and county support for many types of service delivery including health care. Other factors were a rise in the political importance of new groups of poor persons, particularly members of minority populations, who now represented a substantial proportion of all low-income urban residents, and a declining interest in traditional health department services in the face of the explosive growth of therapeutic medicine.

These unpropitious trends all point to a lessening, if not a loss, of the capability of municipal government to continue to discharge its historic role as provider of last report for the health care of the urban poor. The MHSP represented a direct challenge to this perception, and (more positively) the conclusion by the Robert Wood Johnson Foundation that, in fact, local government was the agency best positioned to plan and to implement service delivery programs directed to the unfinished business of the Great Society, i.e., more and better care for residents of the inner city. It engaged the leadership of the mayor not only to maintain the current level of health care services but also to improve them in several basic respects: to increase access of the poor; to enlarge the scope of care through the integration of preventive and therapeutic services at the same site; to shift the locus of ambulatory care from the municipal (or county) hospital to primary care centers in the communities where large concentrations of the poor live. Resources constraint was an explicit condition: programmatic goals were to be achieved with little additional resources, rather through the redeployment of existing funding and personnel, principally from the hospital to the centers. Improved continuity of care was also anticipated as a result of the shift from hospital-based to community-based services since patients would always be seen at the center by the same physician, who would continue to treat them when admitted to a hospital.

From the vantage of hindsight, it is apparent that by the latter 1970s the dominant role that the federal government had assumed during the period of the Great Society in expanding and improving health care services to the elderly and the poor was about to change. Threatened by the steady rise in health care costs which he was unable to stem, President Carter reneged on his campaign promise to press for national health insurance. Congress, faced with large deficits, backed away for the first time in almost two decades from any new federal health initiatives. Many state legislatures, in the face of similar pressures, also shifted from an expansionary to a maintenance posture.

The demonstration was still in its build-up phase in the fall of 1980 when Ronald Reagan was elected president on a platform which promised to cut back social welfare expenditures and reduce the scope of the federal government in the nation's economy. Many of the Republican campaign planks were enacted into law shortly after the new administration took office.

If the change in the federal administration was the most conspicuous, it was by no means the only radical change in the environment in which the MHSP was implemented. Proposition 13 was passed by the California legislature in 1978 and was followed in the succeeding months and years by a retreat from their commitment to expanding social welfare programs on the part of many other legislatures stimulated in part by efforts to constrain their outlays for health care services. Large cities were confronted with greatly reduced flows of intergovernmental aid as a result of the budget-cutting proclivities of federal and state government. Such fiscal strictures were exacerbated by the decline in the economy that began late in 1979 and, for all practical purposes, did not start to recover until 1983. The MHSP had, altogether unexpectedly, to operate in an environment in which the trend of governmental funding underwent a reversal from expansion to contraction at the same time that localities found their tax revenues diminished by the largest and most severe recession since the 1930s and the numbers of poor people in need of services correspondingly increased.

Fortunately, authorization by HCFA of the Medicare and Medicaid waivers went a considerable distance to insulate the demonstration from the turnabout in government financing for health care. The momentum of government retrenchment was somewhat moderated after the first year of the Reagan administration by congressional opposition to additional cuts directed at the poor and the elderly. Many state legislatures likewise moved more circumspectly when it came to second- and third-year reductions aimed at eliminating health care services for the poor.

In one respect, however, the changed environment contributed positively to the course of the demonstration. The physician pipeline which had been forcibly expanded throughout the 1970s finally produced a sufficiently enlarged output that the clinics experienced relatively little difficulty recruiting physician staff. It should be recalled that an important goal of the program was to compensate for the absence of practitioners in poverty areas partly through the employment of nonphysician personnel. The much looser labor market made it easier for the clinics to hire medical and other types of professional and technical personnel on a full-time or part-time basis, including dentists, nurses, physician assistants, and technicians.

This brief excursion into the sudden radical changes in the political setting within which the demonstration was carried out is a potent reminder that no matter how carefully a social experiment is planned and how well it is executed, the margin for success or failure may reside not in the quality of the plans and in their execution but rather in the stability of the environment—whether it continues supportive, or neutral, or becomes hostile or unfavorable. In the case of MHSP, the environment turned distinctly and unexpectedly adverse. Perusing the following chapters, the reader must bear in mind that over and above the difficulties embedded in local politics and local health care institutions that each demonstration had to surmount, the program leadership also had to contend with a worsening political and economic environment which reduced the total flow of health care dollars available for the poor at the same time that it increased the size of the population in need of public services.

2

The Demonstration in Action

This chapter will describe the history of Municipal Health Services Program (MHSP) implementation in each of the five participating cities. The first section will present an outline of each city's commitments and a description of the actual services that were established.

Although all five cities proposed to build upon existing public health and public hospital resources to expand the availability of comprehensive primary care services for target populations living in underserved neighborhoods, each city's model was unique in program structure and objectives and in local environmental influences. The commitments contained in each city's proposal will be described below.

Baltimore proposed to establish four health centers, each offering comprehensive ambulatory care services, in southeast Baltimore, a predominantly white, ethnic, working-class section of the city which had not benefited from earlier federal neighborhood health center or categorical programs. Although a categorical public health clinic and its satellite which provided limited services had functioned in the target area, community residents generally had not used public sector health services, including the city hospital, despite their proximity. Rather, residents relied upon private physicians and nearby voluntary hospitals for care. Two centers were to be developed by expanding the small, traditional public health clinics, and another two were to be new entities. All of the health centers were to be administered by the department of health, and the budget of the MHSP was part of the health department's budget. All nonphysician personnel were to be hired and all purchasing was to be carried out through the health department's established procedures. The unique feature of Baltimore's program was the designation of a private physician group, the Chesapeake Physicians Professional Association (CPPA), as contractor to staff the health centers, with strong backup ties to the Baltimore City Hospitals, which CPPA also staffed under contract. (The CPPA group was replaced as MHSP contractor midway through the demonstration. An alternative group, the Central Maryland Medical Group (CMMG), succeeded it.)

Cincinnati's public health department was unique among the five cities in that it already was responsible for a network of primary care clinics. These were originally either traditional clinics directly operated by the department or freestanding neighborhood health centers, which ultimately operated under contract from the Cincinnati health department, the designated grantee for all federal and state funds earmarked for the city. Cincinnati proposed to expand services, staffing and hours at two of its clinics and to relocate a third, which was crowded into dilapidated quarters, in a new or renovated facility. However, the real focus of Cincinnati's program was a computerized medical information system which would allow immediate information transfer among all the network clinics and between clinics and Cincinnati General Hospital for specialty and inpatient service referral data. The computerized system was to be developed and implemented by a private consulting firm under contract.

Milwaukee designed the most complex program structure among the five cities. As coordinator the city health department planned to orchestrate delivery of health and social services through an array of independent provider groups located in three shared facilities. The health department would continue to provide its existing package of preventive and categorical services; the county teaching hospital, staffed by its parent private medical school, would provide primary medical care; students and faculty of a private dental school would furnish dental services; a private agency would offer rehabilitation services, and so forth. A public health nurse would "coordinate" the services received by patients from these separate and independent providers, each of which maintained its own administration, billing system, and patient records. The coordinator was to see the patient before referral to a service unit and afterward to complete the patient's MHSP record.

St. Louis proposed to convert two of its categorical public health clinics to comprehensive ambulatory care centers, to relocate a third, and to build one new comprehensive clinic. The proposal called for the department of health and hospitals to establish a new administrative division for ambulatory care and to adapt the traditional categorical clinics to a comprehensive primary care model. St. Louis had a nominally unified health and hospitals agency, but the public hospitals division was never related closely with the health division, which was a traditional, nursing-dominated, categorical agency. Most of the hospital medical staff had little respect for the qualifications and competence of health division physicians. St. Louis was able to reorganize and open four clinics, although one site was soon closed amid a budget crisis with little community opposition.

San Jose, like Milwaukee, developed a proposal which required the city to coordinate the operations of a variety of other participating jurisdictions and agencies. The city had neither a health department nor a hospital, both of which were county functions. The city of San Jose agreed to subcontract with Santa Clara County, whose representative, the director of the county hospital, would act as project director. The county would then further subcontract with two existing community-based clinics, one of which was to expand hours, staff, and services to become an MHSP site, and the other to establish two satellite clinics as MHSP sites. The city's formal control extended only to negotiating the contract with the county and influencing the subcontracts with the community clinics. All subsequent input was of necessity limited to advocacy and lobbying.

Despite a slow start, all five cities succeeded in implementing the required number of clinics or more. The clinics fell into two broad types: preexisting facilities which added staff, services, and/or hours, and new delivery sites which required extensive renovation or new construction before services could be initiated. Each of the five cities included within its program at least one preexisting clinic with plans to expand or reorganize existing services. In most of the cities, the preexisting services were traditional preventive or well-baby clinics operated by the public health department. Other preexisting sites included freestanding community health centers and ambulatory care centers operated by public hospital outpatient departments. The new entities were more difficult to initiate because they required site selection, acquisition, and renovation or construction *de novo*. Completion of the renovation or construction for new clinic sites required from two to five years to accomplish. Table 1.1 shows each city's MHSP clinics by year of initial participation and by prior existence status.

In Baltimore, the first two MHSP sites were two public health clinics with limited prenatal and well-baby services. Center A, in a district health building, was colocated with other city social services and a mayor's advocacy station. Center B, a satellite clinic located in a high-rise housing project, targeted geriatric services to the predominantly elderly residents, and family services to younger households neighboring the high rise. Physicians specializing in internal medicine, pediatrics, and obstetrics/gynecology were rotated through the sites by the private physician group, CPPA. These two sites were in operation by August 1978. However, renovations planned for the larger site were never completed due to a lack of funds. The renovation of a church for Center C and new construction of Center D as part of a commercial complex were completed by May 1981. Center E began operating in a temporary trailer in order to meet the August 1981 deadline for participation in the demonstration. A permanent facility was to be built, but the project encountered repeated delays, and construction had not yet started by late 1983.

Cincinnati initially designated two sites from its 14-clinic Primary Health Care System for the MHSP. Center F was a community-based neighborhood health center operating on contract from the health department.

Table 2.1   MHSP Clinics by City and Year of Initial Participation

City	July 1978-June 1979	July 1979-June 1980	July 1980-June 1981	July 1981-June 1982	July 1982-June 1983
Baltimore	2	2	4	5	5
	Center A*	Center A*	Center A*	Center A*	Center A*
	Center B*	Center B*	Center B*	Center B*	Center B*
			Center C	Center C	Center C
			Center D	Center D	Center D
				Center E	Center E
Cincinnati	2	2	2	4	4
	Center F*	Center F*	Center F*	Center F*	Center F*
	Center G*	Center G*	Center G*	Center G*	Center G*
				Center H*	Center H*
				Center I*	Center I*
Milwaukee	0	3	3	4	3
		Center J*	Center J*	Center J*	
		Center K	Center K	Center K	Center K
		Center L	Center L	Center L	Center L
				Center M	Center M
St. Louis	1	2	4	3	3
	Center N*	Center N*	Center N*	Center N*	Center N*
		Center O*	Center O*	Center O*	Center O*
			Center P		
			Center Q	Center Q	Center Q
San Jose	2	4	3	4	4
	Center R*	Center R*	Center R*	Center R*	Center R*
	Center T	Center T	Center T	Center T	Center T
		Center U	Center U	Center U	Center U
		Center V			
				Center S*	Center S*
Total participating	7	13	16	20	19

Number of preexisting clinics: 11 (one closed)
Number of newly established clinics: 11 (two closed)
Note: An asterisk (*) indicates a preexisting clinic.

Center G was a clinic managed directly by the health department. Since both centers already offered relatively comprehensive primary care, the plan was to expand hours, services, and staffing gradually rather than to create a new service model. A third (and later a fourth) existing site was to be relocated, and extensive renovation or new construction essentially turned these into new clinics. The two initial MHSP sites were actively participating in the program with some expanded services by January 1979, although the clinics had difficulty in recruiting physicians for adult medicine. Cincinnati was unable to resolve community disagreements over where to relocate the other two clinics until late in the program. The new sites, Center H, a renovation, and Center I, a consolidation of clinical services within the health department's new administration building, were not operational until August 1982.

Milwaukee planned to include in the MHSP Center J, a high-volume ambulatory care center operated by the county hospital. Because the structure of the Milwaukee proposal involved the colocation, cooperation, and participation of city, county, state, professional school, and private agency providers, this already operational clinic was not integrated with MHSP until July 1979. Center K introduced a public health preventive services clinic into an old emergency hospital and added primary care and other services in July 1979. Milwaukee also planned to renovate an elementary school building for another new clinic site, Center L. This facility opened in the spring of 1980 with preventive and primary care services available and a plan to phase in the services of other providers over a year as further renovations were completed. Center M, a community health center operated jointly by a community organization and a voluntary hospital and funded under the Urban Health Initiative, was integrated with the MHSP in mid-1981, but the city was not involved in either site selection or renovation.

The St. Louis proposal provided for the utilization of two preexisting sites. Center N was a former Model Cities community health center, which was absorbed by the health division in the early 1970s. It was the only freestanding municipal clinic providing comprehensive primary care services when it was included in the MHSP. Center O, a traditional public health clinic, was to be renovated and reorganized to provide comprehensive family care. Although the program was officially declared operational in October 1978, delays in filling physician and administrative positions meant that truly comprehensive services were not regularly available in both centers until 1979. St. Louis also planned to relocate two former public health clinics in renovated or newly constructed facilities. In order to meet the deadline for opening its two replacement sites, the city used temporary trailer facilities. One trailer site, Center P, was abandoned late in 1981 because of budgetary constraints and political upheaval, but renovation of a funeral home to house Center Q proceeded during 1982, and the site was occupied in June 1983.

In San Jose, the initial proposal stipulated the expansion of limited services at Center R, a preexisting community-run health center, to the specification of a comprehensive model. This addition of hours and staffing was accomplished by January 1979. Later in the course of the demonstration, instability of some provider groups led to a decision to bring in a second preexisting site, Center S, a traditional county-operated categorical clinic. Although this site was not proposed until the third year of the program and officially designated just before the August 1981 deadline for participation, actual implementation as evidenced by hiring of physician and administrative staff was delayed almost another year. San Jose relied upon one community clinic to establish two satellite facilities as MHSP units, plans for each of which were already well advanced. Intended to be part of a series of county-fostered multiservice centers, one satellite, Center T, was established in temporary quarters in March 1979, until the multiservice center could be completed. The other, Center U, was located in the downtown area to serve a "core population" of substance abusers, the mentally ill, and the elderly. The city and county then agreed to allow a second established community clinic to start its own satellite, Center V, thus dividing the service area for the proposed downtown facility with the original provider and expanding the MHSP to four locations. All were operating by mid-1979. Subsequently, the county clinic, Center S, was substituted for the second downtown satellite when it closed due to budget shortfalls.

Service Models Under the MHSP

Services were organized in the MHSP demonstration following a diverse set of models. The ownership and governance of the clinics, the clinic organizational structure, the source of physician and support staff, the relationship to the backup hospital, the ownership of the hospital, and the type of services provided all varied among and within cities. The only city which had a uniform structure for all its clinics was St. Louis, and even there historical differences led to variations in style of practice.

Baltimore's service models came closer than those of any other city to the style of a private group practice. In particular, Center D, a family practice site affiliated with a voluntary community hospital, functioned essentially as a group practice. The remaining four sites, which offered primary care services by a multispecialty physician group and mid-level practitioners, had a closer tie to the public health department. The large Center A, which previously operated as a categorical public health clinic, and its housing project satellite, Center B, had difficulty in shedding its image of a free public health clinic even after comprehensive services were initiated. The two other newly established centers carried less of this legacy but still attracted a large uninsured patient load and collecting payment for services proved problematic.

All of Baltimore's MHSP health centers provided basic primary care services for adults and children, including care related to childbearing. Basic services were provided by the major private physician group at each site, following either a family practice or multispecialty mode. Although only the family practitioners spent all their time at a single site, all staff did generally establish individual relationships with patients, and did admit and follow patients for hospital care. Ophthalmology, optometry, and podiatry were provided part-time at the centers under contract by private practitioners. The two largest centers (A and D) offered all three services, the small satellite (B) only podiatry, and the two medium-size centers (C and E) podiatry and optometry. Dental care was provided at three of the five sites, excluding Centers B and E. Only Center A, the former public health clinic, operated an on-site laboratory which also performed lab work for the satellite. The other three centers had contracts with a private lab. The three largest centers operated radiology services on site, which also served patients referred by Centers B and E. Three of the centers which were affiliated with the health department provided some on-site pharmacy services, but prescriptions were filled by the public hospital pharmacy and picked up at the center later. Two centers were located next to a private pharmacy which served patients at their own expense.

The MHSP centers each made use of a social worker from the public hospital for a half day once a week, but otherwise they concentrated on primary care rather than categorical supportive services. Preventive and educational services were considered the primary care provider's responsibility, rather than separate services to be administered or delivered independently. Public health nursing was not emphasized as much as primary medical and dental care, especially at the three new sites.

Cincinnati proposed to expand existing primary care services at three member clinics of the health department's primary health care system. The budgets of all the clinics, whether city- or community-run, are approved by the health department. Centers F and G, a former federal community health center operated under contract and a categorical clinic, respectively, joined the MHSP at the beginning. While each ostensibly offered comprehensive services, budget shortages and staff turnover produced gaps in primary care services at intervals throughout the life of the program. Center G offered internal medicine, pediatrics, reproductive care, and some on-site dermatology. Dentistry was provided during 1979 but terminated in mid-1980. On-site laboratory and pharmacy services, as well as nutrition and social services, were available. Much emphasis was placed on public health nursing, and nurse contacts represented a large proportion of the clinic work load. This site retained a strong traditional public health flavor despite its preexisting primary care base. The major contribution of the MHSP was a strengthened presence of full-time pediatricians, internists, and family practice physicians.

Center F offered adult medicine (both internal medicine and family practice), pediatrics, and reproductive care, as well as dentistry, allergy, psychiatry, radiology, and laboratory services on-site. A private pharmacist was a tenant in the building but did not contribute revenue or generate costs to the program. The National Health Service Corps provided dental and medical personnel at this center. Occasionally both dental and obstetrical services were unavailable due to staff turnover or maternity leave. This clinic relied less on nursing services, reflecting its community health center origin.

Two additional public health clinics were added to the MHSP late in the program. Delays in selecting new sites meant that the clinics did not open in their new locations until late summer and fall of 1982. Center I had previously offered only prenatal, family planning, and pediatric services, and added adult medicine when it was merged with a sexually transmitted disease clinic. It also offered laboratory and pharmacy services; nevertheless, it remained heavily reliant on public health nursing activities. Center H had provided the basic primary care medical specialties, as well as part-time ophthalmology and optometry. It also provided dentistry, laboratory, and pharmacy services, as well as nutrition and social services. Radiology was referred to the central health department facility. Public health nursing was a major service here as well.

Public health nurses were responsible for triage, patient education, immunization, and counseling. Most patients who were treated by a physician also were seen by a nurse. The definition of mid-level practitioner was quite broad in Cincinnati, and many reported visits were probably not for medical diagnosis and treatment, services which could be considered a substitute for physician care. Since Ohio does not authorize practice by mid-level providers, their role as physician substitutes is problematic. Some outside criticism by physicians in Cincinnati was reported in relation to assuring adequate supervision of mid-level providers, but the clinic staff seemed to work well together.

Milwaukee designed the most complex program model among the five cities. Of its four clinics, Center J was a well-established, large ambulatory care facility operated as a downtown outpost by the suburban county hospital. Centers K and L were new sites set up under the MHSP, and Center M was a privately owned health center funded by the federal Urban Health Initiative and affiliated with a voluntary hospital and a community organization. The city health department's plan involved colocation of services provided by several agencies at each of the sites. The three public sites were to offer primary care services provided by physician staff of the Medical College of Wisconsin and support staff from the county hospital, mental health services by the county mental health complex, income maintenance and social services by the county department of social services, and preventive care by the family health project of the municipal health department. Two sites, K and L, also offered physical therapy provided by an agency called Curative Workshop and dentistry provided by students from Marquette University School of Dentistry. Municipal preventive services were also to be provided at Center M, which offered its own primary care and children's dental screening services. The centerpiece of the Milwaukee model was the creation of the new role of service coordinator to tie together all the diverse services.

The primary care component was established at the three public sites utilizing internists and pediatricians; the private clinic also employed a family practitioner. Laboratory services were provided at all sites. Only

Center J offered radiology; it served as the referral center for the other public clinics until it closed in 1981. It also had the only on-site pharmacy. The other clinics wrote prescriptions to be filled by private pharmacies or by the county hospital. The mental health, physical therapy, and social services components were established as planned but had little interaction with the primary care and dental services.

The nurse service coordinator's role was not well defined at the beginning of the program. It was an awkward position to assume because it implied responsibility for making decisions about the services patients were to receive from several independent providers and controlling the flow of information about services and patients. In the case of primary care services, this meant that public health nurses were perceived as infringing on the professional domain of medical school faculty and hospital-affiliated nursing and administrative staff. There was suspicion and resentment from the beginning: county staff would not share medical records with the service coordinators, nor would they refer patients for an encounter to which they attached no value. For months after it opened, the private clinic declined to allow the nurse coordinators to occupy any of its limited office space and was otherwise uncooperative. The municipal health department steadfastly maintained its interest in providing preventive services only and the public health nursing division was allotted the majority of staff positions funded under the MHSP, while the providers of primary medical care, mainly county employees, became more and more estranged from the program. Within the health department, introduction of the service coordinator was viewed as a successful new undertaking; however, outside observers viewed the role as irrelevant to the direct provision of services or were simply uninformed as to what the service coordinators were supposed to to. Most patients interviewed at the MHSP sites were not aware of the service coordinators and did not use them.[1] Their role in the delivery of primary health care was probably negligible.

St. Louis modified services at two of its public health clinics, relocated another, and added one new site to provide comprehensive primary care services. Center N had previously been a comprehensive Model Cities health center and Centers O and P had been categorical maternal and child health clinics in the traditional public health mold. These latter two clinics (Center P subsequently was closed) underwent a major change in philosophy in which the historic dominance of public health nursing was replaced by a medical model of primary care. A great deal of conflict was engendered between the traditional public health nursing staff and the new administrators who wanted to implement broader physician responsibility and services, and this led to the resignation of a number of nurses and termination of the public health nurse training activities which had long been carried out in the health division. The clinics still had to rely on many per-performance physicians but were able to recruit some full-time staff after the city eliminated a $25,000 salary ceiling in 1981.

Each clinic provided multispecialty primary care in internal medicine, pediatrics, and obstetrics/gynecology. The two largest sites, Centers N and

O, also offered dentistry and some ophthalmologic care by resident physicians from a nonuniversity-affiliated residency program at the municipal hospital. These centers also included on-site laboratory, radiology, and pharmacy services, as well as social services, health education, outreach, and specific prenatal and family planning programs. The former Model Cities clinic, Center N, also provided mental health services. Centers P and Q operated in temporary trailer facilities, and Center P, which was relocated from an old public health clinic, was open for less than a year. Their support services were more limited, but they did provide social services and limited laboratory services, and referred patients to other MHSP centers for radiology and dentistry. City budget cuts led to interruptions in denture and vision care services at Center O during the program.

The St. Louis MHSP sites, while still retaining a distinct identity as public clinics, changed their predemonstration focus most thoroughly of all the cities' clinics. They were required to undergo a greater transformation to meet the goal of comprehensive primary care than were the clinics of other cities. To some degree, establishing new clinics (Baltimore, San Jose) or expanding sites which already offered primary care services (Cincinnati) was easier than relinquishing traditional approaches as St. Louis had to do.

San Jose proposed a structure which involved complex interrelationships among multiple governmental levels and community organizations but simple clinic service models. At first, three clinics were to be included. A small community clinic, Center R, was to expand to evening and Saturday hours with the funds from the MHSP grant. A large neighborhood health center was to use MHSP resources along with Urban Health Initiative funds to establish a satellite, Center T, for comprehensive primary care in an underserved community. A third site was to be established in San Jose's downtown area to serve the "core population," including drug abusers, the mentally ill, and infirm elderly patients. Both parent health centers, already participants in the MHSP, wanted to sponsor the downtown site. Competition was strong enough that eventually two clinics were approved, each to be a satellite of one of the parent centers. Center V, the satellite associated with the smaller parent center, was to serve mainly families with an emphasis on maternal and child care. Center U, a second satellite associated with the large neighborhood health center, was to address the needs of older adults and the "core population."

Center R added evening and Saturday services, including general medicine and dental services, with on-site laboratory and radiology and some nutrition, outreach, maternal and child health, family planning, and mental health services. A limited pharmacy was maintained, but generally patients were responsible for having prescriptions filled at private pharmacies.

Center V, a satellite of Center R, offered mainly pediatric care with some general medicine. Obstetrics patients from both clinics were referred to a voluntary hospital under an agreement for prenatal care and delivery at a reduced rate. Dentistry, mental health, and radiology services were provided at the parent clinic, where all dental and mental health records remained. Most laboratory work was done on-site, and prescriptions were filled by private pharmacies. This satellite clinic closed in April 1981, and was replaced by Center S, a former county hospital satellite clinic.

Center S had offered primary pediatric and maternity-related services, with some general medicine. Also provided were on-site dermatology and otolaryngology, as well as dentistry, laboratory, radiology, and pharmacy services. The clinic was staffed by part-time physicians from the county hospital. The major change instituted under MHSP auspices was stabilization of physician staffing with more full-time employees.

The large neighborhood health center was parent to the two other MHSP satellites. Center T, a comprehensive clinic, offered a full range of primary care services, including internal medicine, pediatrics, obstetrics/gynecology, family practice, and dentistry, as well as general surgery. Laboratory, radiology, and pharmacy services were provided on-site, as well as social services, health education, outreach, and mental health services. Center U, designed to serve the "core population," provided internal medicine and general practice (for children and mothers), dentistry, optometry, laboratory, pharmacy, and nutrition services. Both satellites had fairly large support staffs, reflecting the wide service array and generous staffing of the parent clinic, a neighborhood health center on the early model established by the Office of Economic Opportunity (OEO).

Physicians at the San Jose MHSP clinics were employees of the community health centers which operated the clinics and were not, except in the case of the county clinic, affiliated with the public hospital. The staff of Center R did not have admitting privileges at community hospitals, but physicians at Centers T and U could admit at several voluntary hospitals (and in fact had financial incentives to do so). San Jose was the only city where no public health department participated in the MHSP and thus categorical preventive services were not a part of the model.

All the participating cities were able to provide the required range of services. Their delivery styles ranged from a model very close to private practice, to a neighborhood health center, to a modified public health clinic, though all offered at least basic general medical care for adults and children. By September 1983, the national program managers reported that the criterion of providing on-site health care for at least 50 hours per week was met by only three clinics in San Jose.[2] This criterion, considered important early in the program and met by six sites a year earlier, was pursued less vigorously as the result of low off-hours utilization and high costs per visit.

Staffing Patterns

Field research associates surveyed the organization and staffing patterns of all the MHSP clinics in 1980 and 1981, a mid-demonstration period when most sites were in operation. The description that follows is drawn from this survey of nineteen operating clinics. All data are for calendar year 1981, except in the case of Cincinnati (calendar year 1980) and San Jose (July 1980 to June 1981). The total number of full-time equivalent (FTE) employees associated with the MHSP ranged from 66 in Cincinnati to 203 in Milwaukee (including all program components—see Table 1.2). The number of central administrative staff employees for each city ranged from 3.6 FTEs in San Jose to 21.9 in Milwaukee. Milwaukee employed the largest number of doctors and dentists, 20.3 FTEs, and Cincinnati the fewest, 10.5. No city used a large number of mid-level practitioners. St. Louis had the largest contingent with 6.8 FTEs, and Milwaukee and Cincinnati the smallest, each with 3.0 FTE mid-level providers.

Individual clinics varied widely in staff size from nine to 75 employees with a mean number of 29 employees per clinic. The number of physicians and dentists ranged from only one-half FTE to 7.5 FTEs per clinic, with a mean of 3.7 FTEs. Mid-level practitioners, used in 16 of the 19 clinics surveyed, ranged from one-half to four FTEs, with a mean of 1.5 FTEs.

The proportion of medical service providers (defined as physicians, dentists, and mid-level practitioners) among total clinic staff also varied greatly from clinic to clinic, ranging from under 10 percent (in Center P in St. Louis) to 39 percent (in Center D in Baltimore). Former traditional public health clinics generally had a small complement of providers (under 20 percent), as exemplified by the St. Louis centers and Center A in Baltimore. Except for its private sector Center M, Milwaukee's clinics had few providers relative to the large numbers of nurses and support personnel (reflecting the variety of nonmedical services provided in the Milwaukee model). Clinics that approximated group practices in their operations, especially those in Baltimore, showed lower ratios of support staff to providers. These were new health centers, which hired only essential support staff, and there was no legacy from an earlier model to perpetuate. In San Jose, the two smaller clinics had a high proportion of providers, because at Center R the MHSP contributed only staff members required to expand evening hours, and at Center V, which had a brief life span, most support functions were provided by a parent clinic. The two more extensive sites were satellites of a large multifunctional community health center based on the model of early Office of Economic Opportunity (OEO) clinics, and had high levels of administrative and other support staff. Cincinnati's clinics had moderately

Table 2.2   Full-time Equivalent MHSP Employees by City and Category

Employee category	Baltimore	Cincinnati	Milwaukee	St. Louis	San Jose
Total staff	93	66	203	157	100
Central administrative	11	5	21.9	18.8	3.6
Physicians, dentists	14.9	10.5	20.3	11.3	13.3
Mid-level practitioners	3.6	3.0	3.0	6.8	6.0
Support staff	63.5	47.5	157.8	120.1	77.1

high proportions of providers, reflecting a pre-MHSP shift to primary care. Cincinnati's Center F, which had originated as a federal community health center, had the city's highest ratio of provider to support staff. In general, larger clinics had higher concentrations of such medical support personnel as laboratory, radiology, and pharmacy staff, and often extended these services to smaller clinics whose scale of operations did not justify their inclusion.

Because in most of the MHSP target areas ethnic minority groups represent large proportions of the population, it was of interest to ascertain the extent to which clinic staffing contained members of ethnic minorities. In Baltimore, where the target area consisted of predominantly white neighborhoods, about three-quarters of the clinic staff (at four sites from which data were available) were white, one-quarter were black, and a tiny proportion were Asian. Baltimore had three black providers (physician, dentist, or mid-level practitioner) among its staff. Administrators were predominantly white. About 80 percent of patients at these clinics were white, although one small site served predominantly black clients (about 75 percent) and another had a 30 percent black clientele.

Cincinnati's three clinics showed an overall equal distribution between black and white staff. Seventy percent of providers were white, 15 percent were black, and there was one member each of Hispanic, Asian, and other ethnic groups. At Center F, the former OEO clinic, 75 percent of administrators were black, while all were white at the other two clinics. The patient population at Center H was 92 percent white, at Center F, 90 percent black, and at Center G, three-quarters black to one-quarter white, patterns which somewhat approximated the ethnicity of each clinic's staff.

In three Milwaukee sites for which data were available (all but Center M, the private clinic), whites constituted 71 percent of the clinic staff, blacks 21 percent, and Hispanics 8 percent. Milwaukee was the only city in which all of the providers at the time of the survey were white. Subsequently, services at Center L in a predominantly black neighborhood have been provided by a private group of black physicians. The Hispanic support staff are mainly employed at Center K which serves a predominantly Spanish-speaking community.

St. Louis served predominantly black neighborhoods at Centers N and Q and a mixed, primarily white community at Center O. Sixty-eight percent of the St. Louis MHSP staff were black, but 78 percent of the providers were white, 13 percent were black, and 9 percent from other ethnic categories (not Hispanic or Asian). Support staff reflected the ethnic patterns of clinic clients: the highest proportion of white staff worked at the clinic at which 85 percent of visits were from white patients.

Staff at the two San Jose clinics for which data were available was broadly representative of the several ethnic groups found in the population. Sixty-four percent were Hispanic (predominantly Chicano), 23 percent were white, 9 percent were Asian and 7 percent were black. Among providers, blacks accounted for 14 percent and the three other groups were evenly distributed at about 29 percent each. Less than 10 percent of the patients seen at the two clinics were black and Vietnamese, and the balance was fairly evenly divided between whites and Chicanos.

The MHSP clinics' overall staffing patterns seem to reflect hiring of personnel from the ethnic groups served by the clinics, although not necessarily in proportion to their numbers. Professionals have been predominantly white. Black employees are particularly likely to hold nursing or clerical jobs, except in San Jose, where Hispanics are likely to hold these positions.

MID-LEVEL PRACTITIONERS

Although mid-level practitioners were employed at 16 of the 19 MHSP sites operating in 1981, their impact on service delivery and especially on costs to payers was not as great as the program goals envisioned. This is partly due to the fact that state certification requirements and practice codes for mid-level providers and reimbursement for their services were not supportive in three of the states where the MHSP was implemented—Ohio, Missouri, and Wisconsin. During the demonstration period, Ohio and Missouri issued rulings on medical and nurse practice that were overtly antagonistic to any substitutive role for mid-level practitioners in the performance of physician services. Diagnosis and treatment by nonphysicians were prohibited in these states. The rulings evoked sufficient concern about liability for malpractice on the part of nurse practitioners working in Cincinnati's MHSP as to suggest the possibility of moving out of the state. Missouri's ruling against nurse practitioners raised serious fears in the St. Louis Ambulatory Care Division about its ability to continue to use nurses for the large volume of well-child and family planning services they provide.

The second major factor limiting the expanded use of mid-level practitioners was the lack of support and, in some cases, antagonism of some clinic physicians. St. Louis and Cincinnati were the sites where there was explicit physician criticism, but clinic administrators were able to devise protocols for supervision by other staff physicians to counter the specific complaints. Baltimore's family practice model clinic did not support use of mid-level practitioners, but they were employed by the multispecialty group at the other four Baltimore clinics. The strongest collaboration was in the obstetrics/gynecology service, where a nurse-midwife was an equal partner with the physician staff in caring for all patients. St. Louis also used a nurse-midwife at Center N, but neither the midwife nor the physician staff could perform deliveries at the city hospital because none had admitting privileges. In contrast, the Baltimore team had arrangements to admit and deliver patients at Baltimore City Hospitals.

In all five MHSP cities, mid-level practitioners functioned in conformity with written protocols and general, if not specific, physician supervision, in that a physician was required to initial the patient's chart after the mid-level practitioner had completed the needed care. No mid-level providers practiced independently, although at times physician supervision was by telephone rather than on-site. No mid-level practitioners could prescribe medication. Services were billed as though a physician had provided the care.

Baltimore, St. Louis, and San Jose made the most extensive use of mid-level providers. In Baltimore and St. Louis, the explicit rationale was that they were less expensive than physicians, an especially serious considera-tion for low-volume clinics where the cost of staffing all primary care ser-vices with pediatrician, internist, and obstetrician personnel was prohibi-tive. Nearly all the mid-level providers were nurse practitioners (family, pediatric, family planning, or adult) and nurse-midwives, rather than physi-cian assistants (used in Center B in Baltimore). Mid-level providers who were working in former federal community health centers appeared to have somewhat more expanded roles in diagnosis and treatment or ongoing patient management than those in former traditional public health clinics. In some of the latter clinics, nurse practitioners were required to spend up to half their time in traditional nursing tasks, or followed protocols limited to preventive services rather than the diagnosis and treatment of acute or chronic illness.

The Medicare and Medicaid waivers were not reported to have had any positive effect on the use of mid-level practitioners or on how their services were billed or reimbursed. Milwaukee's attempts to secure Medicare and Medicaid reimbursement for preventive services by public health nurses have not been successful, and the lack of state support for nurse practition-ers was a major barrier to implementation of the Medicare waiver for preventive services in Milwaukee.

Utilization of the Clinics

The MHSP clinics in all five cities experienced slow growth in utilization during the early stages of the program. Projections of visit volume in the cities' grant proposals generally overestimated both the total utilization and the rate at which use would increase. Staffing (particularly physician staffing in Baltimore and primary care and dental staffing in Milwaukee) was planned for higher volumes of patients, and the desultory rise in work load produced high unit costs early in the program. This in turn created a need to adjust staffing levels downward, leading, at some clinics, to prob-lems in providing the full range of primary specialty services other than on a part-time basis. In most clinics, visit volume did not increase rapidly until 1981, year three of the project. Substantial growth continued through 1982 and 1983.

The rate at which patient utilization of the MHSP clinics developed is partly related to the proportion of new versus expanded clinics. Preexisting clinics started from an established base. The new sites, however, generally did not become operational until after an extended period spent in site location, renovation or construction, and staff recruitment. The number of preexisting clinics ranged from one each in Milwaukee and San Jose (which added a second, older clinic late in the program) to all four in Cincinnati (although the two designated for relocation were not included as official participants until the relocations were nearly completed). Table 1.3 shows base-year work load, projected and actual incremental visits for the pro-

Table 2.3   MHSP Utilization by City, Base-Year Actual, Projected and
Actual Annual Increment, Final Year

City	Base-year work load	Projected annual incremental visits by final program year[1]	Actual annual incremental visits by fifth program year	Total annual visits by fifth program year (1982-83)
Baltimore	4,419	101,295	90,948	95,367
Cincinnati	36,355[4]	28,450	81,050[2]	117,405[2]
Milwaukee	42,600[3]	28,000	52,103	52,103
St. Louis	26,236	153,812	51,359	77,775
San Jose	33,974[4]	83,855	74,816	108,790
Total	143,584	395,412	350,276	451,440

Notes: [1] Incremental visit projections were taken from each city's original grant
proposal.
[2] A large proportion of Cincinnati's reported visits are encounters with
nurses only.
[3] Milwaukee's only preexisting clinic, which was its largest volume site,
closed late in 1981. Thus, no base-year visits appear in year five.
[4] Cincinnati and San Jose brought older, preexisting clinics into the program
in the fourth program year. Their visits are included as base-year work load.

Source: Carl J. Schramm and Gary A. Christopherson, Final Annual Report to the
National Advisory Board, Robert Wood Johnson Foundation Municipal
Health Services Program, 1983.

gram. The base-year work load of the existing clinics was not recognized by
the Johnson Foundation toward earning grant funds; only incremental
visits were counted. Base-year work load ranged from 4,419 visits in Baltimore to 42,600 visits in Milwaukee. For the total demonstration, Cincinnati and Milwaukee planned modest increments of about 28,000 annual
visits by year five, while the other cities were much more ambitious. St.
Louis' projected increment of 153,812 visits by the final program year
proved to be unrealistic. However, according to the annual report of the
national MHSP administration, by the end of the fifth year incremental
annual visits ranged from 52,103 in Milwaukee to 117,405 in Cincinnati,
although a large percentage of Cincinnati's were simply public health nursing visits.[3] The reported visits include not only physician and dentist services but all types of ancillary and preventive services as well. Growth was
slow during the first three years, with the largest boosts from the addition of
new sites rather than expansion of older clinics. During the fourth and fifth
years, visits increased dramatically in all five cities.

   Baltimore and San Jose successfully marketed the enhanced package of
Medicare services to the elderly population beginning early in the demons-

tration and sites offering dentistry experienced surges in Medicare utilization. Milwaukee and St. Louis began marketing later and their efforts drew a somewhat less significant response by these groups which grew more rapidly in the fourth and fifth years. Cincinnati did not market the Medicare services for four years; ultimately a number of uncoordinated efforts yielded some results. In Cincinnati, the elderly contributed a disproportionately low number of visits relative to the total work load of the program.

Not unexpectedly, growth in incremental utilization suffered setbacks in the three cities where clinics had to be closed. The largest Milwaukee site, which provided over 42,000 visits per year, was closed in late 1981 during the third year of the program in order to reduce the county hospital's operating deficit. St. Louis relocated a former public health clinic to a temporary trailer site, Center P, in an abrupt and little publicized move to cut operating costs; a few months later, during the program's third year, services at the trailer were terminated. Only the temporary site had been considered part of the MHSP, and it had been very sparsely attended as a result of its abrupt initiation. San Jose lost one of its satellite clinics, Center V, when start-up costs overtaxed the capacity of the parent facility, Center R. Center V, which had provided about 6,000 visits a year, was discontinued early in the fourth year of the program.

The low initial use of the MHSP sites probably implies that there was no severe lack of access to medical care in the target neighborhoods, at least at a threshold below which only aggressive outreach and case finding would succeed in bringing unserved patients into the system. The sluggish growth may also reflect the need of public health clinics to overcome their traditional image as places where patients could receive only categorical services and as resources intended only for the poor. Privately insured patients did not enroll in the clinics in large numbers, but uninsured patients did. The consistent growth over time indicates that the services apparently were acceptable to those who used them. The range of services available was definitely expanded, and new services were used particularly by the Medicare population.

Utilization data were reported quarterly to the Robert Wood Johnson Foundation by the city project directors, noting patient visits by provider type, age and sex, and registration status. Data from these reports are the basis for this analysis; there are, however, some caveats about their use. In many cases, there are internal inconsistencies in the patient visit figures, and often quarterly figures vary from reported annual totals. Rather large discrepancies are found in month-to-month patterns of volume by provider type in individual clinics or single cities, and apparently the criteria for distinguishing among nursing visits, other support staff visits (such as pharmacist or nutritionist), and actual mid-level practitioner (certified nurse practitioner or physician assistant) visits differed from city to city. Cincinnati, Milwaukee, and St. Louis reported large numbers of mid-level practitioner visits in which the services performed were actually more in the nature of public health nursing than medical diagnosis and treatment. Many were traditional public health nursing functions: family planning, prenatal, well-child, and immunization services.

Additional utilization information was collected directly from the individual clinics by field research associates. Clinic and health department record keeping and reporting mechanisms were found to produce numerous inconsistencies. In many cases, a clinic system generated two or three conflicting counts of the number and types of services provided, depending upon the purpose for each set of data. Billing reports thus often differed from appointment logs or from totals generated for such divisional reports as nursing activities and family planning services. It is important, therefore, to use utilization data discriminately, to be cautious about drawing conclusions from small categories of information, and generally to look at trends rather than absolute numbers. Especially in clinics where the MHSP is but one element in a larger array of programs, reporting of MHSP-related activity may show extensive variation from source to source.

BALTIMORE

Baltimore converted a health department clinic, which provided fewer than 4,500 annual child health visits, into an MHSP site, Center A. All other utilization was added under MHSP auspices. Center A maintained about the same volume of services during the first project year, though it shifted to greater use of physicians and more adult medicine. Visit volume doubled during the second year, with the greatest growth in pediatric and maternal services. During the third year, Center A reached almost four times its original work load, doubling the adult medicine utilization from the previous year, and adding dentistry. Specialty services (podiatry, ophthalmology, etc.) also increased dramatically. While pediatrics and maternity care stabilized, adult medicine, dentistry, and specialty services continued to grow rapidly into the fourth year, reaching over 24,000 visits, 90 percent of which were to physicians or dentists.

Center B, a small housing project outpost, provided about 2,000 visits in the first program year, added about 1,000 visits per year thereafter, reaching over 5,000 annually. Growth was most pronounced during early 1982, the latest period for which data are available. Adult medicine was the most extensively used service at the satellite because of the high elderly population at the housing project, and about one-half of these patients were cared for by a physician assistant. The full-time mid-level practitioner was more appropriate for this low-volume site than maintaining full-time both an internist and a pediatrician.

Center C, which was established in the spring of 1981 in a converted church, grew rapidly, adding about 1,000 visits each quarter to reach an annual rate of over 20,000 visits by mid-1982. General medicine generated about one-quarter of these visits to a mid-level practitioner, but the largest number of visits was to other providers such as podiatrists (over 5,600 in FY 1982), optometrists, ophthalmologists, and dental hygienists. Dental visits totalled almost 2,000 for the year ending in mid-1982.

In July 1981, Center E began operating in a temporary trailer site. During its first three quarters it doubled its visit volume each successive reporting period, but growth slowed in the fourth quarter, the last for which data are available. The first year's work load was just over 3,600 visits, about one-half of which were provided by mid-level practitioners, particularly the general adult medicine services. About 20 percent of the visits were to a pediatrician and about one-quarter were for obstetrics/gynecology services.

The fifth Baltimore clinic, Center D, was a family practice site that opened in the spring of 1981. Its work load grew over five-fold from its first quarter to June 1982. A little less than half the 18,000 FY 1982 visits were to family practice physicians, over one-third were to dentists and hygienists, and most of the balance were for vision care and podiatry.

During calendar year 1981, Baltimore's clinics showed a wide range of provider productivity. According to field associate data, visits per physician/dentist ranged from 456 to 4,280 at Baltimore's MHSP sites. Visits per mid-level practitioner ranged from 438 to 1,477. Total visits per FTE employee (all staff) ranged from 138 to 696. The highest volume clinics showed the highest productivity; the newest site showed the lowest. The clinics were required to meet productivity criteria established by the national program managers. Work load and staffing figures were adjusted to account for the start-up needed to build volume. As reported in October 1982, none of Baltimore's clinics met the criteria of 4,500 visits per physician and 2,250 visits per mid-level practitioner before adjusting for the start-up factor, but three of the five conformed to the adjusted guideline.[4]

Baltimore's clinics generally showed slow growth or stabilization in utilization by children and adolescents. High rates of growth were apparent for the elderly, attributable to the Medicare waiver and its marketing, with elderly women outnumbering elderly men. Use by females in the reproductive years also grew steadily. Adult males were much lower users, but their visits also increased steadily.

Baltimore placed greater emphasis on marketing its MHSP program than any other city, and did so earlier in the implementation process. The project director hired a marketing specialist who concentrated first on the Medicare population and then on local business and industrial employers for health contracts. A substantial work load buildup, especially in services to the elderly, can be attributed to Baltimore's marketing efforts, which began in earnest with a study in the spring of 1980 which recommended changing the program's image to that of a group practice and hiring a marketing specialist. A change in the contract physician group at this time also contributed to increased marketability and productivity.

Baltimore's first two MHSP clinics had about a 30 percent rate of missed appointments at the beginning of the program. Center A reduced the rate to about 20 percent by early 1982, but the no-show frequency remained high at Center B. The two new large health centers, C and D, were able to maintain no-show rates below 15 percent, compared to Center E with a rate of over 20 percent. All sites except Center B experienced continuing large gains from new registrants. This satellite apparently drew clientele only from the limited area of the housing project.

CINCINNATI

Cincinnati's MHSP project brought on board two preexisting clinics as of January 1979. Each had previously provided from 7,000 to 8,000 visits a year, most of which were concentrated in pediatric care. Center G offered traditional public health services while Center F, a neighborhood health center, operated under a health department contract. The quarterly utilization data show erratic visit patterns by specialty area and provider type, indicating that from quarter to quarter, separation of physician visits from nurse visits may have been inconsistent. Cincinnati's definition of mid-level practitioner is not as specific as Baltimore's and San Jose's, where state guidelines regulate the certification and scope of practice of physician extenders. Visits to nurses are not specifically identified, while some visits reported as mid-level are in fact to nurses, nutritionists, WIC workers, social workers, and similar categorical personnel. These caveats are particularly important in assessing the data from the clinics operated directly by the health department.

Center F reported fairly constant utilization over the course of the project, ranging from just over 14,000 visits during 1979 to just under 14,000 in 1981. During the second quarter of 1982, mid-level provider visits increased, while physician visits declined dramatically in adult medicine and obstetrics/gynecology due to staff turnover. Pediatrics represented a steady proportion of work load (25 percent) throughout the project, and dentistry contributed under 1,000 visits per year. This clinic failed to attract large numbers of the elderly, but utilization was fairly balanced between males and females, especially for children and adolescents. Adult males and the elderly contributed the lowest proportion of visits. No group showed significant increases in utilization.

Utilization at Center G dropped during the first three quarters of 1979 to about half its original quarterly volume, and then resumed a slow but steady growth. Excluding one anomalous figure from the first quarterly report, the trend in visits to physicians doubled from about 1,300 per quarter to an average of 2,600 per quarter in mid-1982. The reported visits to mid-level practitioners showed erratic decreases and increases in the first two years, and growth from an annual rate of about 4,000 in 1980 to a quarterly rate of over 4,500 early in 1982. Since there was less than one-half FTE mid-level provider reported on the staff, it is difficult to reconcile these figures. The physician visits were almost evenly divided between general adult medicine (45 percent) and pediatric services (35 percent) with the remaining 20 percent in obstetrics/gynecology. Distribution of the reported mid-level visits is not clear. Center G continued to focus on care for children and mothers, and while services to adults increased, they were provided primarily to women. Use by the elderly rose only slightly and remained a small fraction of the annual work load of about 27,000 visits in FY 1982.

Centers H and I, originally a health department clinic which offered some adult medicine, and a child health, family planning, and sexually transmitted disease clinic, respectively, joined the MHSP in July 1981, although they were not actually located in their permanent quarters until August 1982. Center I provided a reported 18,416 visits between July 1981 and July 1982, 32 percent of which were physician visits, mostly pediatric and maternity. Only a handful were from elderly patients or adult males. A similar pattern was reflected in reported utilization figures for Center H, where pediatric and maternity-related services represented well over half of the 23,000 to 28,000 visits in the first year of operation. Dentistry contributed about 10 percent of the visits. By the last reported quarter, nonphysician visits totalled almost two-thirds of the work load, and as no mid-level provider staffing was reported, it must be assumed that these visits were mostly to nurses. Fertility-related and pediatric visits predominated, with only a few visits from elderly patients.

Cincinnati's health department had a clear policy not to compete with private providers, and hence engaged in very limited marketing, with little emphasis on attracting patients by the offer of expanded benefits under the Medicare waiver. The clinics retained a strong identity as public services, with little resemblance to group practice. Although an appointment system was introduced, data were not available on the rate of missed appointments, a reflection of the predominance of nursing rather than physician services. Except at Center F, most physicians were employed part-time.

Calculating productivity figures for Cincinnati's MHSP clinics is difficult because of the problems in identifying the visits attributable to various types of staff. Figures collected by a field associate researcher for calendar year 1980 indicated physician/dentist productivity ranging from just over 2,500 to just over 4,100 visits at the sites for which data are available. Visits per FTE employee (all staff included) ranged from 764 to 1,071. Physician/ dentist productivity, actual and adjusted for the start-up factor, was reported by the national MHSP program managers in late 1982 to met program criteria in three of four sites.[5]

MILWAUKEE

The first Milwaukee site to join the MHSP, Center J, was a large downtown outpost of the county hospital which had been in operation for several years, providing about 40,000 visits a year in a multispecialty clinic setting. It included a large walk-in unit and a smaller primary care division which used full-time personal physicians for continuing basic medical services. The municipal health department added a separate preventive health component which provided under 1,000 visits a year, with a fairly stable quarterly work load. The primary care work load decreased by a little over 10 percent per quarter over the life of the project until the clinic was closed at the end of 1981. The entire primary care work load was handled by physicians, with the vast majority of visits in adult medicine. About 30 percent of appointments were missed.

Two new clinics were established with primary care services provided by the county hospital, prevention by the health department, dentistry by a local dental school, and rehabilitation services by a private agency. Center K began operating in July 1979. During its first year, dentistry and preventive services represented the lion's share of the approximately 6,700 visits recorded. Primary care was added at the end of the year but even during FY 1982 it contributed only about 3,600 visits, almost all in adult medicine. By 1982, the last year for which data are available, dentistry visits had grown to almost 5,000 with constant quarterly increases, rehabilitation visits had leveled off at 1,400, vision care visits (added in late 1981) were growing dramatically (over 1,100 of a total of 1,600 visits for the year took place in the last quarter), and preventive services had risen to almost 4,400 visits per year and were also still increasing. The annual total for all services was over 16,000 visits.

The other new site sponsored by the health department, Center L, began operating in the spring of 1980 offering dentistry and preventive services. Dentistry grew in the first year by 400 to 500 visits a quarter, and generally maintained this trend until a surge to almost 600 visits in the second quarter of 1982. Preventive services contributed from about 650 to about 1,200 visits a quarter until a reported 4,000 visits in the second quarter of 1982. Vision care was added in the spring of 1982 and accounted for approximately 200 visits. Primary care, mainly adult medicine, contributed just under 1,500 quarterly visits by mid-1982, showing a steady growth curve, and doubling during the second full year of operation. Total reported visits reached 15,885 for FY 1982, less than a third in primary care, almost 45 percent in prevention, and the remainder divided between dentistry and rehabilitation. Prevention services are primarily public health nursing services, those traditionally provided by the health department and encompassed by its "Project Life" activities which concentrate on hypertension screening, breast cancer screening, and other categorical services. Missed appointments were very high, 50 percent in dentistry and almost 40 percent in primary care.

Center M was operated by a community group in cooperation with a voluntary hospital. Reported operations began in July 1981 and work load totalled over 10,500 visits for the first year with irregular utilization growth patterns. The third quarter's work load dropped to less than a third of the second quarter's visits, then quadrupled in the fourth quarter. Dentistry contributed about 1,500 visits. Physician visits accounted for 75 percent and mid-level practitioner visits for 25 percent of the 9,000 primary care visits. Pediatrics constituted about a third of visits and the balance were in adult medicine, family practice, and maternity care. Only 135 preventive visits were reported for the year. Missed appointments were reported at about 25 percent.

Data collected by a field research associate for 1981 indicated a wide range of physician/dentist productivity in Milwaukee's MHSP sites, from 491 at a two-month old clinic to 5,675 at Center J. Visits per FTE employee (all categories) ranged from 156 to 589. The national program managers reported in late 1982 that one of Milwaukee's sites had reached the established productivity criteria of 4,500 visits per physician and 2,250 per mid-level practitioner after adjusting for the start-up factor.[6]

The three Milwaukee clinics which survived into 1982 still attracted large numbers of new registrants, although reported figures showed some inconsistencies. The elderly had begun to increase their use of dental and vision care services covered under the Medicare waiver at the two clinics for which data are available. The loss of Milwaukee's largest site, Center J, meant that citywide utilization was cut approximately in half, but the three remaining clinics continued to grow in the 1982–83 period.

Milwaukee began marketing its MHSP in 1981 and 1982 through public service announcements and meetings with community groups. Public awareness of the MHSP was limited, however, partly because of the combination of many independent provider groups which maintained their separate identities, partly because of the location of the project administration as a small component of the health department, and partly because political leadership was essentially unaware of the program—the mayor's interest lay with preventive services under the "Project Life" title. Thus marketing efforts were low-key and did not have much visible impact.

ST. LOUIS

The two St. Louis sites which joined the MHSP as established clinics were Center N, a former Model Cities comprehensive health center operated by the health division, and Center O, a traditional categorical health clinic. Center N increased its work load from 6,650 visits in its first quarter to over 10,200 visits in the second quarter of 1982. The annual rate of utilization grew from under 30,000 in 1979 to about 40,000 in 1982. The designation of physician and mid-level practitioner visits is not completely clear, although a group of nurse practitioners who worked at Center N were transferred to the city hospital in 1981, partly due to lack of legal support by the state of Missouri for physician extenders. Based on reported data, mid-level practitioners provided more than half the visits at Center N until they were transferred. However, for billing purposes, all visits were reported as physician visits. Dentistry contributed about 7,000 visits a year, although the quarterly work load in mid-1982 had reached an annual rate of over 10,000 visits. Medical visits, which were concentrated in pediatrics and fertility-related care early in the program, were fairly evenly balanced among those specialties and adult medicine by mid-1982.

Center O almost doubled its quarterly work load from mid-1979 to mid-1982, referable to an increase in pediatric and obstetrics/gynecology services, to about 1,800 to 2,000 quarterly visits each, and the addition of adult medicine which contributed about 2,200 visits quarterly. Total work load was over 28,000 visits for 1982, the last full year for which data are available, including dentistry, which represented almost a quarter of the patient volume.

The two other St. Louis sites were both located in temporary trailer facilities during the period for which utilization data are available. Center P was open for only three quarters, during which it provided a total of about 2,200 visits, primarily pediatric and prenatal visits carried over from categorical services previously offered at a nearby public health clinic which was closed. Fewer than 100 visits were provided to the elderly, who had been considered the largest market for this clinic. Center Q, which began operating late in 1980, grew fairly consistently to about 2,500 visits per quarter by the middle of 1982. About 50 percent of the visits were in obstetrics/ gynecology, while another third were in pediatrics, and the balance in adult medicine. In mid-1983, this site moved into permanent quarters, a renovated building in a neighborhood with little available medical care and a growing population, and is likely to have experienced rapid growth since then.

St. Louis' clinics reported fairly high missed-appointment rates, from about 20 to 35 percent, over the course of the project, without apparent changes over time. Center O showed a large and growing utilization by the elderly and continued growth in pediatric and fertility-related utilization as well. Center Q had low use by the elderly and high use by maternal and child health patients. Center N showed a preponderant patient load of women in their childbearing years and of children, although use by the elderly also grew, especially among females. All of these utilization trends matched the predominant sociodemographic patterns of the neighborhoods surrounding the MHSP clinics.

Productivity at St. Louis' MHSP clinics ranged from 4,639 to 5,381 visits per physician/dentist in 1981. Total visits per FTE employee (all categories) ranged from 820 to 999. Data for two clinics are excluded because of inadequate information. The national program managers reported in late 1982 that two of the three St. Louis MHSP sites met program productivity criteria in both absolute terms and after adjustment for the start-up factor.[7]

St. Louis, suffering from severe city and health services budget shortfalls, was able to invest little in marketing. Public service announcements, speaking engagements with community groups, and distribution of leaflets were probably responsible for some of the increase in utilization by the elderly under the Medicare waiver, especially at the converted categorical clinic.

SAN JOSE

San Jose sponsored five clinics in the course of the MHSP. One clinic, Center V, closed during 1981 and was replaced by Center S. Data for these two sites are somewhat sketchy and are limited to the periods for which they were functioning.

Center V, a satellite of Center R, operated for just over a year and a half, beginning in the fall of 1979. It offered adult medicine and pediatric services in about equal volume, and reached an annual rate of some 6,000 visits by the time it closed in the spring of 1981. On its termination, this clinic was replaced by an off-site outpatient facility operated by the county hospital, Center S. Utilization data are available only for two quarters, and these figures reflect previous patterns of service delivery of about 25,000 visits a year, over a third in adult medicine, 10 percent in obstetrics/ gynecology, half in pediatrics, and the remainder in subspecialties such as dermatology, podiatry, and otolaryngology. No trend data are available for this site.

Center R financed evening and weekend services through the MHSP. It added about 500 visits during its first quarter and more than tripled this volume by the end of 1981, the last quarter for which data are available. About half the visits were for dental services, and the rest were in family practice, with mid-level practitioners providing almost half these services. About 6,300 visits were provided in 1981. In late 1982, the weekday clinic was included in the MHSP but no data are available on its utilization.

The other two San Jose clinics were satellites of a large neighborhood health center. Center T, planned as a comprehensive family primary care clinic, began operating early in 1979. During its first year it provided about 5,000 visits but reached an annualized rate of almost 12,000 by the last quarter. During 1980 it provided over 13,000 visits, and in 1981, almost 30,000. Over a quarter of the visits were for dental services, and dental utilization, much of it by Medicare recipients, grew steadily and strongly. About a quarter of the primary care visits were provided by mid-level practitioners. Obstetrics/gynecology represented a fairly small proportion of visits, but some pediatric and fertility-related care was provided by family practitioners. The elderly were a large factor in utilization from fairly early in the project, and males represented about 40 percent of patients overall, in contrast to other cities' experience.

Center U, located in the downtown area to serve a "core population" of severely disadvantaged patients, also drew heavily on the elderly population. Starting operations late in 1979, it quickly drew a clientele for dentistry (1,500 to 1,800 visits a quarter) and family practice/adult medicine. Annual utilization was about 20,500 visits in 1980 and 21,600 in 1981. Mid-level practitioners served about 10 percent of the work load. Optometry contributed about 1,000 visits a quarter by 1981. Growth was slow but continuing at the end of 1981, the last period for which data are available.

San Jose's clinics indicated a fairly low missed-appointment rate of under 15 percent. Productivity, as reflected in data for FY 1981, ranged from 1,173 to 2,724 visits per physician/dentist and from 955 to 3,436 visits per mid-level practitioner at the four clinics then in operation. Visits per FTE employee (all staff included) ranged from 276 to 715. The national program managers reported late in 1982 that one of four clinics met program productivity criteria before adjustment and three of four met the guidelines after adjustment for the start-up factor.[8]

Marketing as an overall program activity was fairly limited, partly due to the structure of the San Jose MHSP, with multiple subcontractors for services delivery, and to conflicts among subcontractors and the city/county administrators of the program during 1981 and 1982. These disputes occupied the attention of administrators, providers, and community advisory groups and make any marketing efforts virtually impossible during the period.

Quality of Care

A clinically oriented assessment of the quality of care provided by the MHSP clinics was beyond the scope of this evaluation. The issue of quality is addressed instead through a number of proxy indicators related to the staff and the service models, and through the expressed opinion of local political, professional, and community leaders. Information was collected about the credentials and training of the physician staff of the clinics as one indicator of quality. Characteristics of high quality ambulatory care such as comprehensiveness and continuity can be ascertained from descriptions of the scope of services and the referral arrangements for specialty and inpatient care. The physical amenities of the clinic facilities also lend an element of quality, affecting the perceptions of patients and staff alike. Another indicator of a clinic's concern with quality is the existence of formal procedures for medical chart audit or some other quality review. In general, it appears that by most of these proxy measures, the quality of care, and certainly its accessibility, were improved by the MHSP in its target neighborhoods. The circumstances in each city will be discussed briefly.

BALTIMORE

From the inception of the Baltimore MHSP, all physician staffing was provided through contracts with private physician groups. The initial group were all faculty members at Johns Hopkins University School of Medicine and had admitting privileges at Baltimore City Hospitals. This group was later replaced by a competing multispecialty group which staffed four of the clinics and a family practice group which staffed one. All physician members of these two groups were board certified or eligible in their respective specialties, all were graduates of American medical schools, and most had recently completed their training. None were over age 60, and none engaged in independent private practice outside the group, although they did not spend all their time in practice at a single clinic. Baltimore's physician groups each had quality assessment or medical audit committees and procedures to maintain high-quality care.

Baltimore's clinics offered comprehensive primary care services, and continuity of care was assured by the ability of the physicians to admit and follow patients. Continuity was not based on the clinic's relationship with a single back-up hospital but on the relationship of individual physicians with one or more hospitals, including the public facility (especially for obstetrics patients) and numerous voluntary institutions.

Physical amenities varied in quality. The family practice site, Clinic D, was located in an attractive new facility. Clinic B, the housing project satellite, operated in cramped, ill-designed quarters. Limited renovations had made modest progress in changing the image of Clinic A, the former categorical clinic. The renovated church, Clinic C, was bright and pleasant but awkwardly laid out for health services, and the trailer in which Clinic E was located had predictable drawbacks, which will no doubt be improved by eventual construction of a new facility. As the majority of sites for care were new, the MHSP clearly expanded access.

The public's perception of quality of care at the MHSP centers was apparently very positive. The physician groups who provided services had uniformly favorable reputations among patients and the community. Local leaders offered praise and raised no criticism of the quality of services. Medical professionals also were generally favorable in their comments about the MHSP health centers.

CINCINNATI

Cincinnati's health department hired the physicians and dentists for its directly operated health clinics. Among 14 individuals assigned to the two clinics for which data were available, only two worked full-time in the clinic. All were board certified or eligible, three were foreign medical graduates, and four were aged 60 years or older. Three of the staff were in private practice. At the contract neighborhood health center, three of five staff members were full-time and the others half-time employees. All were board certified or eligible, none were either foreign medical graduates or over 60 years old, and two were in private practice. Three staff members were assigned through the National Health Service Corps. The health department administered centrally established quality assurance and medical audit procedures for all clinics.

Cincinnati's MHSP sites offered relatively comprehensive primary care, although some clinics went through periods when no staff member was available in one of the primary care specialties due to a hiring freeze or to staff turnover. Continuity was less than ideal because physicians generally could only refer patients to the public medical center and could not admit and treat inpatients. The health commissioner made a strong effort to secure closer ties between the medical center and the clinics and was able to get approval for admitting privileges but not in hospital supervision of patients for clinic physicians.

Two of Cincinnati's clinics, Clinics H and I, obtained new or renovated facilities with much-improved physical amenities over the course of the project. Clinic F was located in a fairly new building, but Clinic G maintained an aura of the old-fashioned public health clinic with limited comforts.

While public support for the health department's clinics has remained high, the services are perceived as intended not for persons with the ability to pay for care but for the poor or medically indigent. The quality of care is not openly criticized, but it is perceived as characteristic of a public facility of last resort. Local leaders consider services to be of generally high quality and believe the health commissioner has continued to improve the quality and efficiency of the clinic's operations. The teaching hospital's medical leadership has been sufficiently impressed with the upgrading of clinic medical staff that limited admitting privileges for clinic physicians have been approved.

MILWAUKEE

One of Milwaukee's MHSP sites, Clinic M, was staffed entirely by physicians from the National Health Service Corps. All were full-time employees, newly trained in American schools, and board certified or eligible. None had independent private practices. In the other three sites, at the time the information was collected, the medical staff was provided through the county hospital by the local medical school. About one-third were board certified or eligible, one-third were foreign medical graduates, and one person was aged 60 or over. All staff at the two smaller new clinics were part-time employees, while at the large county-operated site over half were full-time. A separate component provided mental health services through the county mental health center with approximately one full-time psychiatrist at each of the three public centers. Dental services were provided at the two smaller sites by faculty and students from a local dental school, with part-time staff each present for only a half day a week. The dental clinics were teaching facilities, and nearly all 20 to 25 supervising dentists at each site were in private practice as well.

Each of Milwaukee's MHSP clinics offered a very comprehensive range of services in a single facility but the services were essentially provided independently of one another and not much interaction among provider groups took place. The county-affiliated physicians were able to admit and follow patients at the county hospital and physicians at the private clinic could do the same at the affiliated voluntary hospital. Although a new private physician group replaced county staff at one site, continuity of care was maintained because the individual physicians had full admitting privileges at one or more of the various inner-city voluntary hospitals. No program-wide quality assurance program was in place for the Milwaukee MHSP, although staff were planning to develop such procedures during 1983.

The clinics in Milwaukee distinguished themselves both in terms of physical facilities and quality of care. The three public clinics were housed in public buildings (two former municipal hospitals and one elementary school) which were spacious (ranging from 27,000 to 40,000 square feet), characterized by fine woodwork and elegant appointments, and located off the main thoroughfares. The two clinics which were opened for the first time were remodeled with purpose and clientele clearly in mind: services are color-coded, signs are visual as well as verbal, and waiting and treatment rooms are sunny, cheerful, and noninstitutional. The private clinic with its more limited range of services is located in a smaller and less attractive buillding which, nonetheless, was built as a private medical office facility and would not offend middle-class consumers.

The quality of care has never been questioned at any of the clinics and is, in fact, assumed by all to be of the level of excellence associated with the sponsoring institutions. Under the original arrangement with the county, all physician staff placed at the clinics held faculty appointments at the Medical College of Wisconsin. The private clinic was staffed by National Health Service Corps physicians selected from the residents trained at the sponsoring voluntary hospital. Under neither plan was care provided by students. The credentials of the physicians in the recently instituted minority physician group, particularly the group's leadership, are no less reputable. Despite considerable ill-feeling surrounding bureaucratic arrangements and agreements, the various participants have acknowledged uniformly high levels of competence and motivation on the part of the medical teams.

ST. LOUIS

The medical staff for St. Louis' MHSP clinics were employed by the health division, most of them on a per-performance basis, which meant for two-, three- or four-hour sessions as needed. The majority of the per-performance physicians were private practitioners who supplemented their income by working in the clinic for a limited amount of time. The two larger St. Louis Clinics, N and O, each had one full-time physician in internal medicine and in pediatrics and a half-time dentist, supplemented by several per-performance physicians each week. Staffing varied from week to week. Clinic Q had only per-performance physicians, although its staff was to expand when the permanent facility was completed. More than half the physicians were board certified or eligible, a third to a half had been trained in foreign medical schools, and about a third were aged 60 years or older. Characteristics varied depending upon which local physicians worked at any given time.

The fact that so many different physicians were employed meant that a continuing doctor/patient relationship was difficult to establish. Continuity also suffered because clinic physicians did not have admitting privileges at the public hospital. Formal referral mechanisms for inpatient and specialty care were weak, although they began to improve by the end of the project. The clinics offered a comprehensive range of primary care services, which greatly expanded the previous service mix.

Clinic N operated in a large neighborhood health-center facility constructed with Model Cities' money several years before the MHSP was launched. While the facility was perhaps larger than the current work load warranted, it was attractive and comfortable with many amenities such as public meeting rooms and attractive furnishings. Clinic Q was to be located in a totally renovated building and was planned with patient comfort and attractiveness in mind. Clinic O operated in an old public health building ill designed for primary care practice which had received modest refurbishing and more and better equipment, but which still lacked such basic amenities as an elevator.

In St. Louis, like Milwaukee, no program-wide quality assurance procedure for the MHSP was in place. Public opinion about quality of care in the MHSP sites varied according to the interest group queried. Community leaders in the neighborhoods affected were uniformly positive in their comments on care at the clinics. Health division staff were also generally of the opinion that the care provided was a good quality and had improved from the earlier period. Those affiliated with the city hospital, a teaching facility, were critical of both the cost and quality of care at the centers, reflecting the persistent hostility between the health and hospital bureaucracies in St. Louis. The medical society's representative gave a generally positive report. Representatives of public health nursing and maternal and child health services felt that although a good medical model of service had been instituted, the counseling, home visiting, and other public health nursing services had deteriorated, lowering overall quality. Most community organizations were very supportive of the program. Many community leaders and center staff felt that the clinics had lower costs than the outpatient department (OPD), but a number of health professionals thought that the clinics cost as much as the OPD. Most professional and political leaders who were questioned believed the city could not afford to continue operating all the clinics when the grant ended.

SAN JOSE

Data on medical staff characteristics were available only for two of San Jose's MHSP clinics. All physicians were board certified or eligible, none were over 60 years old, and none were foreign medical graduates. Only one was a full-time employee, and most of the part-time staff were also in private practice. A comprehensive range of primary care services was provided. Physicians had full admitting privileges at the public county hospital or at one of several voluntary hospitals near the clinics, and continuity was thus assured via the affiliations of the individual physicians rather than through fixed program or clinic procedures. Established quality assurance mechanisms were not in place, which led to criticism of the management of some of the clinics by the community in the course of the demonstration.

The facilities at three of the sites were relatively new, while Clinic R was housed in an old building that had once been a parish hall. The latter was physically cramped, dingy, and poorly designed for the provision of health services. That clinic had posited as its highest priority the attainment of a physical plant on a par with the other MHSP clinics.

Opinions about the quality of health care provided by the various MHSP clinics were far from uniform. It was noted, however, that on one objective measure, stability of staff, all of the clinics except the county site were deficient, having suffered significant staff turnover during the project. This frequent shifting of employees was partly a result of internal dissension over the proper management of services and partly due to the instability of the various sources of funding upon which the clinics depended. Frequent professional staff turnover is likely to have a negative impact on the continuity of care, which is one component of quality. The community advisory groups for Clinics T and U raised serious questions about the quality of care provided at their clinics. An array of federal and state agencies responded to these criticisms by investigating the parent health center as well as the two satellites and found numerous deficiencies in the ability of the clinics to provide satisfactory services. However, these agencies, persuaded that sufficient progress in correcting the problems had been made, approved the continuation of their funding for limited periods of time under stringent reporting conditions. The issue of quality of care became highly politicized at the two large satellite clinics. Although some of the criticism was justified, it is probable that the issue was exaggerated in the heat of the contention among the community factions involved. Leaders who were unaligned with either faction were reluctant to express any opinion about the quality of care.

The smaller clinic and its satellite were not as closely scrutinized. The frequent turnover in the director's position (seven incumbents in two years) affected professional staff stability. The staff were considered by most local leaders familiar with the program to be basically qualified with potential for improvement. Less uncertainty about future funding might have enabled the clinic to improve its physical facilities and equipment, which would also have contributed to enhanced quality of services. The quality of care was not a politicized issue here as it was at the other clinics.

Notes

1. Dario Albert Rozas, "Dichotomous Client Utilization Patterns in Milwaukee's Experimental Neighborhood Health Centers," in Scott Smith and M. Venkatesan, editors, *Advanced Health Care Research* (Provo, Utah: Brigham Young University Press, 1983).

2. Carl J. Schramm and Gray A. Christopherson, *Municipal Health Services Program: Final Annual Report 1982–83* (The Robert Wood Johnson Foundation, October 1983).

3. Ibid.

4. Ibid., 14

5. Ibid., 15

6. Ibid., 16

7. Ibid., 17

8. Ibid., 19

3

Resources

The previous chapter revealed the wide diversity in MHSP implementation by examining the commitments and accomplishments of each of the five participating cities. This chapter will continue that discussion in the context of program costs, revenue structure, and transfer of resources.

Program Costs

The Municipal Health Services Program was to be built upon existing public health and hospital resources. The private grant dollars were added to current health department or community clinic operating budgets, budgets which derived their revenues from a variety of sources, including patient and third-party billings, state and federal grants, city or county cash or in-kind subsidies, contractual agreements, and so forth. The MHSP and the individual clinics included under its auspices were required to segregate their financial accounts from those of the parent agency responsible for program implementation so that program costs and revenues could be monitored. The implementing agencies were further required to establish mechanisms to bill patients or their insurers for services and to collect all available revenues in order to achieve financial viability on termination of grant support at the end of the five-year demonstration period.

In four of the five cities, the MHSP budget was placed under the umbrella of the municipal health department. The majority of participating clinics in Cincinnati and St. Louis were preexisting public health clinics or community health centers operated through the health department. All operating costs of these clinics were considered MHSP costs, including a variety of public health activities that were also supported by categorical grants and local subsidies. Health department administrative costs were not generally allocated to the clinics, although the specific administrative costs associated with MHSP implementation and authorized by the grant were reported and paid for. In Baltimore and Milwaukee, the MHSP clinics were essentially new enterprises with a separate identity from other health department activities. Each of these two cities brought into the MHSP private or other public service providers, either as independent collaborators or under contractual agreements. The clinic budgets for one city thus were comprised of a number of separate, independent cost centers that were merely colocated in a single facility. Each participating provider constituted an independent financial entity. In the other city, all the basic primary care services were covered by the program's budget, but ancillary or specialty services at some of the sites were furnished by independent contractors who rented space; their operating costs were not considered part of the program budget. In San Jose, the MHSP was structurally located within the county hospital, to which its administrative costs were allocated. However, services were provided by independent community health centers that operated as subcontractors; each of these had activities, costs, and revenues that were not considered part of the MHSP, but nevertheless contributed administrative support to the MHSP clinic operations.

The previous description serves to indicate the complexity and intricacy of defining MHSP program costs, even before attempting to address the adequacy or appropriateness of the financial accounting systems employed by the public agencies that participated in the demonstration. It is questionable whether the variable structure of the program from city to city, the often disparate strategies for allocating agency costs among clinics, and the likelihood of differences in defining the boundaries of the MHSP within the parent agency(ies) permit valid comparisons of costs across clinics or across cities. The nature of the cost and revenue data reported and the inconsistency among multiple sources of data for each element suggest caution in drawing any conclusions about the true cost of providing services under the MHSP or the relative costs of clinic care and hospital outpatient services. The quality, consistency, and specificity of the cost data available do not permit firm conclusions. This having been noted, general summary and trend data on program costs will be presented.

BALTIMORE

Total expenditures for the MHSP rose from an infinitesimal $90,420 in FY 1979 to $4,663,423 in FY 1982, or 9.9 percent of the health department budget. The city subsidy to the MHSP in FY 1982 is estimated at $65,000, compared to the reduction of $2,746,843 in the city subsidy to the health department between 1978 and 1982. Baltimore has been very successful in substituting state and, to a lesser degree, private dollars for local and federal support to its health department.[1]

Baltimore's MHSP clinics provided about 65,700 visits in FY 1982 at a unit cost of just over $68, excluding central administrative costs. The individual clinics had unit costs ranging from $55 at the smallest site to $87 at the family practice site, which provided a very large volume of Medicare dental services. Cost per visit was initially very high (as much as $180 in the early quarters) for each newly established clinic but decreased steadily as volume grew. At preexisting Clinic A, cost per visit fluctuated, with 1982 unit costs still somewhat below those of 1978–79.

Compensation for physicians, dentists, and mid-level practitioners was equal to about 28 percent of total expenses by FY 1982. Among the five clinics it ranged from 26 to 35 percent of expenses, and was highest at the two smallest sites. Practitioner wages tended to decrease as a proportion of expenses over time as visit volume grew. Personnel costs accounted for from 44 to 69 percent of operating expenses in calendar year 1981 at Baltimore's five MHSP clinics. Over the course of the demonstration, it is roughly estimated that $1.2 million was spent on construction, renovation, and equipment for the five clinic sites, from Urban Development Action Grants, city resources, Urban Health Initiative funds, Community Development Agency contributions, and other sources. Most of these capital costs are not reflected in the operating expenses and unit costs analyzed above.

In FY 1982, the estimated cost per visit at Baltimore's public hospital was $137.94. All the MHSP clinics in Baltimore met the program criterion of maintaining a cost per visit not to exceed two-thirds of the municipal hospital's cost per visit, according to calculations by the national program managers.[2]

CINCINNATI

Total expenditures for Cincinnati's MHSP rose from $1,522,218 in FY 1980 (earliest available data) to $3,465,132 in FY 1982. The complete network of primary care clinics represented a growing proportion of the health department's budget, rising from 32 percent in FY 1977 to 40 percent in FY 1981, as total costs increased by 89 percent during this period.

Cincinnati's four MHSP clinics provided a total of about 90,000 visits in FY 1982 at a cost of a little under $27 per visit, excluding central program administration. The cost per visit at the individual clinics ranged from $25.99 to $32.01. The low cost per visit in Cincinnati is attributable to the large number of visits to public health nurses for traditional preventive services. The cost per visit at Cincinnati's former neighborhood health center, Clinic F, went up about 25 percent in 1980 to $40, but by mid-1982 it had dropped to its 1979 level of $30. The cost per visit at the three other MHSP sites showed a decreasing trend over time. At Clinic G, the unit cost dropped by almost 50 percent from 1979 to 1982. The two remaining clinics joined the project in mid-1981; one showed decreasing unit costs over the year but the other followed an unstable pattern.

Compensation for physicians, dentists, and mid-level practitioners (as defined for salary purposes) totalled about 20 percent of program expenses in FY 1982. Among the four clinics, provider compensation as a proportion of total expenses ranged from 13 percent at Clinic F to 23 percent at two of the others. Trends over time showed no clear pattern. Salaries and fringe benefits accounted for over 75 percent of expenditures at Clinics F and G, as reported by a field research associate for calendar year 1980, and more recent data from quarterly financial reports show a similar citywide pattern, with personnel costs representing from 42 to 82 percent of individual clinic expenses. Nearly all staff are directly employed by the clinics, in contrast to Baltimore, where contractual arrangements for specialty and ancillary services place those costs outside the clinic personnel category.

A rough estimate indicates that about $912,000 was spent on clinic construction, renovation, and equipment in Cincinnati. In addition, development and implementation of the computerized information system received substantial support from MHSP funds, although a precise dollar amount cannot be fixed. Implementation delays and cost overruns plagued the information system, with problems at their height in 1978 and 1979. By 1981 the budget allocation for this function had been reduced some 35 percent from its 1978 level and more progress was achieved, following replacement of the consultant who had been engaged during the early phase with in-house personnel. The information system costs at individual clinics represented up to half of all nonpersonnel expenditures in 1982.

In FY 1982, Cincinnati's MHSP clinics all reported a cost per visit far below the criterion of two-thirds or less than the estimated Cincinnati public hospital outpatient cost per visit of $116.60.[3]

MILWAUKEE

The MHSP clinics in Milwaukee provided a total of almost 58,000 visits in FY 1982. Had the largest clinic not been discontinued in December 1981, the number would have been close to 80,000. Citywide, the cost per visit averaged $57, while the unit cost at individual clinics ranged from $44 to $81. The highest cost per visit was found at Clinic J, which subsequently closed. The intensity of services provided at this site, similar in style to a teaching hospital outpatient department, and a steady drop in utilization over three years meant that even the high volume of visits could not keep costs down; rather, unit costs increased. Clinics K and L, which had high unit costs when they opened ($75 to $90 per visit), were able to reduce the cost per visit fairly consistently over time. Clinic M showed erratic unit cost patterns from quarter to quarter; this may be the result of unreliable reporting of utilization and/or costs.

The proportion of total expenses which was allocated to compensation for physicians, dentists, and mid-level practitioners ranged from 28 to 34 percent in the three clinics still operating in FY 1982. Figures for Clinic J were not reliable. No clear trends were apparent for this measure over time. Personnel costs were responsible in FY 1982 for about 73 percent of total expenditures for the three surviving MHSP clinics. At the individual clinics, personnel costs showed almost no variation from this average. Approximately $1 million—in addition to an undetermined amount of in-kind contributions—was expended on construction, renovation, and equipment for the Milwaukee clinics over the course of the MHSP demonstration.

In FY 1982, the Milwaukee sites all met the criterion of a cost per visit less than or equal to two-thirds of the cost per outpatient visit at the public hospital, estimated to be $143.26.[4]

ST. LOUIS

During FY 1982, the three MHSP clinics still operating in St. Louis provided almost 71,000 visits at an average cost per visit of $55. The unit cost at the individual clinics ranged from $47 to $61. Over the demonstration period, the cost per visit at Clinic N increased, especially early in FY 1982, but a surge in utilization in mid-1982 effected some reduction. The unit cost at Clinic O remained at its 1979 level with erratic quarterly rises and falls. Clinic Q started operating at a high cost per visit (well over $100), but this figure declined concomitantly with increasing utilization during the two years of operation prior to the completion of its permanent quarters.

Compensation to physicians, dentists, and mid-level practitioners ranged from 17 to 28 percent of each clinic's operating expenses; it was lowest at Clinic Q and highest at Clinic O. Over time this proportion decreased at Clinic N, rose slightly at Clinic O, and was stable at Clinic Q. Personnel costs represented about 82 percent of total costs at each clinic. A rough estimate indicates that about $1,850,000, including approximately $25,000 in trailer rentals for 1982–83, was allocated to construction, the use of temporary sites, renovation, and equipment for the four MHSP clinics over the full course of the demonstration project.

In FY 1982, the MHSP clinics all met the criterion of a cost per visit equal to or less than two-thirds of the cost of a visit to the outpatient department of the public hospital. However, the estimated hospital cost per visit of $92.60 was only pennies above the unit cost at one of the clinics. St. Louis was reported to have the lowest hospital cost per visit of the five cities in the demonstration project.[5]

SAN JOSE

San Jose's MHSP clinics provided over 92,000 visits in fiscal year 1982, the last period for which data were available, at a cost of approximately $58 a visit. During 1981 five clinics were in operation for at least part of the year. Clinic V closed at the end of April; its replacement, Clinic S, began to report activity as of July 1. The cost per visit at the individual clinics ranged from $37.50 at Clinic R to $59.50 at Clinic S (for six months' operations). Clinic V had a high cost per visit (over $100) during its first year but had reduced the unit cost to about $57 before a budget deficit forced it to be discontinued. The other clinics showed a decrease in average cost per visit from initial high levels, with quarterly fluctuations and an upward trend toward the end of 1981.

Physician, dentist, and mid-level practitioner compensation as a proportion of total operating expenses ranged from 22 percent at Clinic S to 38 percent at Clinic R, where only the evening and weekend services were components of the MHSP. This figure decreased gradually at Clinic R and Clinic U but increased at Clinic T. Personnel costs represented from 60 to 80 percent of total expenditures at Clinics R, T, U, and V during FY 1981, based on data collected by a field research associate. No estimate was available for expenditures on construction, renovation, and equipment for the San Jose MHSP clinics over the course of the project.

In FY 1982, Santa Clara County's public hospital provided outpatient services at an estimated cost per visit of $113.66, as calculated by national MHSP program managers. Thus all San Jose's clinics met the criterion of a cost per visit less than or equal to two-thirds that of the public hospital outpatient department.[6]

Revenues

In most of the cities, the MHSP served to expand existing publicly sponsored health services which were supported primarily by local resources, augmented by state, federal, and other funds. Patients generally had not been charged for the services. The MHSP clinics were required to institute billing and collection procedures in order to receive patient care revenues for services. Sites which had operated as traditional public health clinics historically had provided free care, and, in some cases, staff were reluctant to require patient payment. To establish the information systems necessary to generate bills for patients and third parties, and to monitor collections of accounts receivable was difficult and time consuming. New functions often had to be undertaken by existing clerical staffs, leading to billing delays and high error rates. Nonetheless, third-party revenues increased substantially over the course of the project in former public health clinics, especially in St. Louis, although nonoperating revenue continued to account for a large proportion of the total budget in many clinics in the participating cities. The change from a free-clinic operation to a more businesslike provider model was problematic not only because of philosophical issues and procedural requirements but also because of the array of services provided and the payer mix of the patient clientele. In addition, for any given payer mix, the revenue-generating capacity was dependent upon the reimbursment rates of the various payers. Medicaid, and particularly Medicare waivers, made the reimbursement potential for services covered by these two payers far more advantageous. Some clinics became so dependent upon waiver revenues that the termination of the waivers could mean an adverse shift in financial status.

The experience of field research associates in collecting data from the MHSP clinics on utilization, expenditures, and revenues indicated, as noted above, that different elements of the financial and reporting systems were likely to generate inconsistent information. The University of Chicago

research team, which is evaluating the impact of the MHSP and the waiver demonstration on total utilization and costs of users, found marked inconsistencies in both absolute numbers and trends over time among three data sources on charges for Medicare services under the waiver: quarterly financial reports submitted to the Johnson Foundation, monthly reports filed with HCFA by the clinics that record utilization and/or charges for services provided under the Medicare waiver, and end-of-year financial reports on costs used by HCFA to reconcile payments and clinic costs.[7] The size of these inconsistencies suggests the possibility of lost bills, billing delays, or defects in the billing process. They also indicate that the revenue reported in the quarterly financial reports often far overstates the revenue that can be confirmed as actually billed. Actual collections are not included in the quarterly financial reports.

A study of financial systems and service and payer mix was carried out in 1982 at one clinic in each city by Laventhol and Horwath, certified public accountants.[8] It was found that in general, the procedures to identify and verify third-party coverage and self-pay patient income were inadequate to determine charges. Little effort was made to collect fees from self-pay patients at the time of services. Accounts receivable were found to be inadequately monitored and aged, and third-party bills were not sufficiently tracked to the point of collection. These problems in billing coupled with apparent inconsistencies in the reporting of revenue suggest the need for caution in interpreting the revenue data presented below, which are drawn for the most part from the quarterly financial reports to the Johnson Foundation.

BALTIMORE

Baltimore's five MHSP clinics showed a wide range in the ratio of operating revenues to total expenditures, from 38 percent to 91 percent in FY 1982. The proportion had increased steadily at all the sites except Clinic B, and exceeded 66 percent at three of five clinics. Net operating revenues (less allowances) ranged from 88 to 95 percent of total operating revenues. The MHSP grant covered from 3 to 33 percent of total expenses per clinic in FY 1982, but no clear trend was visible over time. Citywide, nonoperating revenues reportedly covered 24 percent of total expenses in FY 1982, and had generally decreased over time.

Data collected by a field research associate for calendar year 1981 indicated the following distribution of charges by payer: Medicare, 77 percent; Medicaid, 6 percent; private insurance, 1 percent; and self-pay, 15 percent. It was reported that 93 percent of Medicare, 85 percent of Medicaid, 100 percent of private insurance, and 69 percent of self-pay charges were collected. Nonetheless, for this calendar year these data indicate that nonoperating revenues still constituted 42 percent of total revenues. The ratio apparently improved rapidly in 1982. Self-pay collections were proportionately lowest at the former public health sites and highest at the family practice sites.

Efficient financial management at Baltimore's MHSP sites, particularly billing and collections, was hindered by the requirement to employ health department clerical staff who had little training, and by bureaucratic obstacles in hiring and terminating employees. One response of management was to recruit a cadre of volunteer workers from the community to assist in billing and other financial tasks. A 1983 decision by the city to transform the MHSP into an independent corporate entity removed from the health department is expected to enable the program to improve the quality and productivity of its financial clerical staff.

Since the Baltimore MHSP is heavily dependent on the Medicare waiver, its termination would be a serious threat to the program. Much of the waiver utilization is for services not otherwise covered by Medicare, and it is not certain whether patients who visit the clinics for dentistry, podiatry, vision care, and pharmaceuticals will continue to use physician services once these additional services are no longer free.

CINCINNATI

The MHSP clinics in Cincinnati generated total operating revenue to equal approximately half of total expenditures in FY 1982. However, a high proportion of discounts and uncollectibles reduced the relative contribution of operating revenue. Nonoperating revenue including the large municipal subsidy equalled 78 percent of total expenditures. The individual clinics all demonstrated similar ratios of 74 to 79 percent nonoperating revenue to expenditures. The MHSP grant contributed 15 to 18 percent of total expenditures in the two older clinics and 3 to 5 percent in the two added in FY 1982. No clear trend is visible in the proportion of the grant contribution over time. A continuing commitment to providing free preventive public health services financed by local revenues is evident in Cincinnati. While a system of charges has been developed and bills are rendered for many services, the health department has avoided a serious emphasis on collections in the clinics it operates directly; the contract clinics are more aggressive, however, in pursuing revenues. The public health nursing functions which contribute large increments to utilization totals are supported mainly by the municipal subsidy.

Data collected by a field research associate for Clinics F and G in 1980 confirm that charging and collecting for services had yielded revenues equal to only a small proportion of expenses (27 percent), particularly at Clinic G. The data are somewhat limited, but the distribution of payers for reported charges was as follows: Medicare, 3 percent; Medicaid, 47 percent; private insurance, 1 percent; and self-pay, 49 percent. Collectibility for the various payers was 143 percent for Medicare (due to the waiver and/or lags in payment); 68 percent for Medicaid; and 28 percent for private insurance. It is assumed that Medicaid services were billed as mandated at 76 percent of customary charges, a built-in discount. Self-pay charges were discounted by 58 percent before billing and only about 15 percent was ultimately collected. Reported collections amounted to 21 percent of reported expenditures for the year. Detailed information on grant sources by clinic was not available due to a health department policy of centrally pooling grant revenues and distributing them throughout the clinic network on the basis of need.

Cincinnati was in the process of computerizing its financial accounting systems during the MHSP demonstration. When each clinic is equipped with billing and accounts receivable subsystems, the performance of these functions can be expected to improve. However, patient ledgers are still maintained manually. It is important to recognize the influence of department philosophy on its financial operations. Cincinnati's explicit policy is to remain a public sector service and to refrain from competing in any fashion with private providers. Hence no real effort was made to encourage Medicare waiver utilization: of ail the participating cities, the Cincinnati program treats the lowest proportion of Medicare patients, or at least it fails to bill under the waiver for large numbers of services. The Cincinnati MHSP did not encourage expanded utilization of the newly waivered Medicare services, and this is reflected in the charge data.

MILWAUKEE

At the four Milwaukee MHSP clinics which were in operation during FY 1982, total operating revenue ranged from 33 to 113 percent of total expenses. Clinic J, which closed in December 1981, reported the highest ratio of total operating revenues to expenses, and Clinic M the lowest. Net operating revenue at Clinic J was only 63 percent of expenses, however, and collections may have been even lower. As no MHSP grant funds are reported to have been used at this site, figures on total nonoperating revenues represent only 2 percent of expenses and a deficit is apparent. At Clinics K and L, total operating revenues equalled about half of total expenses. For the three clinics which survived, nonoperating revenue was equal to 60 percent of total expenses. The MHSP grant contributed 15 percent overall, and from 7 to 33 percent of each clinic's total budget. The grant contribution appeared to increase over time at one clinic but was not consistent at the other two. Reported operating revenues appeared to increase over time at Clinics K and L. The Milwaukee provider organizations were unable or unwilling to make available information as to payer mix and collections. Data on charges derived from the quarterly financial reports show that the three clinics operating throughout FY 1982 charged from 18 to 39 percent of their bills to Medicaid; from 12 to 47 percent to Medicare; about 12 percent to private insurance; and from 22 to 36 percent to self-pay patients. Information on collections by payer was not available.

Financial management systems did not appear to generate sufficient collections from patient care activities to allow Milwaukee's MHSP clinics to be self-supporting. Reported gaps and lags in submitting bills for services suggest inadequate billing and collection procedures. However, the complex, multiprovider structure of Milwaukee's clinics meant that several separate, independent financial systems were involved, and reporting was as problematic as billing and collections. It must also be remembered that the MHSP sponsor, the Milwaukee health department, placed its primary focus on preventive services which generally cannot be billed to third parties. The department was willing to contribute nonoperating funds to support these preventive public health activities.

ST. LOUIS

The St. Louis MHSP clinics in FY 1982 generated total operating revenues equal to 87 percent of total expenses. Net operating revenues, however, represented only 36 percent of total expenses. At individual clinics, total operating revenues ranged from 82 to 104 percent of costs, and showed a dramatic increase over time. The MHSP grant support contributed from 8 to 42 percent of expenses, with the newest site receiving the highest level of funding. Annual grant support also increased over the course of the project. Data collected from three of the clinics by a field associate provided information on payer mix and collectibility. For calendar year 1981, Medicare represented 32 percent of charges; Medicaid, 60 percent; private insurance, less than 1 percent; and self-pay, 7 percent. St. Louis reportedly collected 155 percent of what it billed to Medicare, reflecting apparent lags in payment for earlier services. Collectibility from Medicaid amounted to 90 percent of billings, which had already been discounted about 30 percent from usual and customary charges; from private insurance it was 80 percent; and from self-pay patients, 17 percent. Clinic O had a better collection record from self-pay patients than did Clinic M (22 percent and 11 percent, respectively). The St. Louis clinics benefited more from the Medicare waiver as the result of its reimbursement for the full cost of services than from an increase in clientele through the offer of special services, although the elderly did seem to be attracted by dentistry and vision care at one of the sites. Since the city did not have the staffing resources needed to provide a large volume of special services such as dentures, the pattern of dramatic increases in Medicare utilization found in Baltimore and San Jose did not occur.

A major problem in the St. Louis billing system was adequately identifying and verifying third-party coverage and eligibility of patients. Many patients who were billed a minimum charge as self-pay might have been eligible for or actually enrolled in Medicaid. However, the target neighborhoods for the St. Louis MHSP were among the poorest in the five cities, and there was little likelihood that the clinics could wean themselves from municipal subsidy even with strengthened billing systems.

SAN JOSE

Citywide, in 1981 total operating revenues were equal to 79 percent of total expenses for the five San Jose clinics operating at least part of the year. The proportion at the individual clinics ranged from 53 percent at Clinic V to 85 percent at Clinic S. Clinics T and U both had total operating revenues equal to or more than 80 percent of expenditures. This measure increased over time at Clinic T, decreased at Clinic U, and was irregular at Clinics R and V. The MHSP grant contribution ranged from 7 to 29 percent of total expenditures and was highest at Clinic V. This contribution decreased proportionately over time at three of four clinics. Nonoperating revenues were responsible for 19 percent of total expenses citywide, with a contribution that ranged from 8 percent at Clinic T to 74 percent at Clinic V. Net operating revenues were reported as over 80 percent of total operating revenues for Clinics T and U but below 58 percent for Clinics R and V, and 66 percent for Clinic S. Data collected by a field research associate indicated that the payer mix according to charges in San Jose's clinics R, T, U, and V in FY 1981 was: Medicare, 53 percent; Medicaid, 18 percent; private insurance, 5 percent; and self-pay, 23 percent. Revenues from a prepaid health plan to Clinics T and U added about 17 percent to the total. Medicare revenues contributed proportionately more to Clinics T and U, where the waivered services were extensively used, and grew over time. Self-pay charges, private insurance, and Medicaid were proportionately more important at Clinics R and V. Collectibility data were not available.

San Jose's MHSP clinics had some financial management problems, particularly in the areas of managing accounts receivable and adequately screening patients to determine payment status and verify third-party coverage. Several public agencies performed investigations of the internal financial management practices of the larger neighborhood health center which was the contractor for two MHSP clinics after criticism was initiated by community groups. While much conflicting evidence was reported, inadequacies were perceived to exist by municipal leaders. In their own audits and reviews, state and federal agencies recommended a number of improvements in management as a condition for continued funding. Errors in financial planning played a major role in the forced closure of Clinic V. High start-up expenses exceeded the cash flow capacity of the parent clinic.

Financial Viability

It is evident that in all five cities, the MHSP clinics have continued to rely upon municipal subsidies and nonoperating revenues from federal, state, and other sources well into the fifth year of the demonstration. The city of Cincinnati has shown a willingness to subsidize its primary care network with a high proportion of municipal resources, although it has closed low-volume clinics, consolidated facilities, and trimmed staff and services. Its MHSP sites are likely to continue as part of the public system, especially since two are located in newly completed facilities. The Medicare waiver was not heavily used in Cincinnati and no Medicaid waiver was initiated, so termination will have little effect. As resources become more strained, local attitudes may change.

St. Louis has trimmed its other public health services significantly during the MHSP demonstration, closing preventive service clinics, closing one MHSP site, and reducing categorical program activities. Although nonoperating revenue is about 60 percent, the remaining MHSP clinics have a good chance of surviving simply because of the need for them, particularly in view of the continuing curtailment of municipal hospital-based health services. The municipal subsidy is likely to be under pressure to shrink, and staff and services may contract, or one or more clinics may close. Loss of the Medicare and Medicaid waivers will hurt the St. Louis clinics financially, and it is likely that whatever public health services and resources St. Louis is able to maintain will be concentrated in these three clinics in the future, especially if the public hospital clinics should be closed.

While the Cincinnati and St. Louis MHSP clinics are protected to an extent by their position as an integral part of their city's health or hospital department's ongoing interests and activities, this is not true for any of the other cities. The future of the Milwaukee program will be determined by the judgments of each of the participating provider agencies as to their ability to finance operations after termination of Medicare and Medicaid waivers and the MHSP grant. Recently, Milwaukee's three clinics have been heavily dependent upon the MHSP grant to support operating expenses (to the extent of one-third to one-half their costs), and it will not be easy to replace both waiver and grant dollars. It is likely that primary care and dentistry services would be most likely to be withdrawn, since the waiver and grant served more to support them than the social services and mental health programs. The Milwaukee health department will probably continue to provide preventive services, which have been its major long-term interest.

San Jose is another city where no single corporate home accommodates the MHSP clinics. Rather, each clinic has an independent parent organization and each must solve the problems of future survival individually. The county-sponsored Clinic S which was integrated with the MHSP late in the life of the project will no doubt continue to operate, but the MHSP has had a minimal relationship to its previous or current operation. Clinic R, which was able to expand services with MHSP funds, has sufficient political support to maintain some local subsidy but may shrink its services to their preexisting scope and scale. The remaining two large clinics will be severely affected by the termination of the Medicare waiver, but the loss of grant dollars will not have nearly as much impact. One clinic has federal Urban Health Initiative funds, and both have good opportunities to participate in state Medi-Cal ambulatory care prepayment plans. The new political climate in California will favor consortial arrangements for Medi-Cal contracts, which the MHSP structure could foster. The clinics also have strong community and local political support, which may help to assure their survival.

Baltimore is perhaps the most interesting demonstration site. All but one of its clinics were created new in communities which were underserved, though they were not Baltimore's poorest neighborhoods. The city was avowedly attempting to reduce its role in the direct delivery of health care during the demonstration period, and it took steps first, to transfer its municipal hospital from public governance to private, and subsequently, to establish the MHSP as an independent corporate undertaking, removing it from the health department bureaucracy. It is likely that the city will be willing to subsidize the program to some degree in the future, but it will probably seek gradually to decrease the amount. Baltimore's greatest problem will be the loss of the Medicare waivers. Medicare charges account for over three-quarters of the MHSP's operating revenues, and a large percentage of this total goes for the special services such as dentistry, vision care, podiatry, and pharmaceuticals which have served as drawing cards for the clinics. Despite aggressive, efficient top management and highly qualified private group physicians, it is impossible to predict how many Medicare patients will continue to use the MHSP clinics after the waiver is terminated, or whether the conventional Medicare reimbursement will generate adequate revenues for the clinics. Probably at least some of the sites will be able to survive independently, but others may fail.

Medicare and Medicaid Waivers

The Municipal Health Services Program as originally conceived by the Johnson Foundation was a demonstration in reforming the service delivery structure. However, just before the program was launched, the Foundation arranged for the participation of the federal Health Care Financing Administration (HCFA) through the authorization of waivers of Medicare and Medicaid regulations governing benefit coverage and methods of reimbursement. HCFA involvement added a new dimension to the demonstration. The rationale for the participation of HCFA in a cooperative research and demonstration project with the Johnson Foundation was the development of a strategy that would simultaneously increase access to better quality primary care and decrease beneficiaries' total health care costs by modifying service delivery and reimbursement mechanisms. It was anticipated that expanded use of a broader range of preventive, diagnostic, and therapeutic services in a less costly neighborhood clinic would reduce the utilization of more expensive inpatient and emergency room services and thus reduce overall costs per person. Community-based ambulatory primary care was to be substituted for hospital services.

The staff of HCFA were authorized to grant waivers of section 222 of the Medicare regulations to "permit coverage of certain currently noncovered services and to eliminate deductible and coinsurance requirements for beneficiaries receiving services at the demonstration sites. The reimbursement procedure which the Medicare program will adopt is to treat the participating health clinics as if they were outpatient hospital departments."[9] Among the otherwise uncovered services which Medicare beneficiaries were to receive with no out-of-pocket charge from the MHSP clinics were general dentistry, dentures, prostheses, immunizations, eyeglasses, vision care, pharmaceuticals, comprehensive physical examinations, mental health services, podiatry, and physical and speech therapy. These services, especially dentistry, eyeglasses and podiatry, were expected to constitute a major drawing card for the clinics. In addition, the elderly were to be attracted by waiving the usual deductible and coinsurance charges.

HCFA invited states to apply for waivers of section 1115 of the Medicaid regulations (the "state-wideness" requirement) to allow the MHSP clinics to be reimbursed by Medicaid in the same way as provided by the Medicare waivers: as hospital outpatient departments on a retrospective full-cost basis. States were also allowed to request waivers of Medicaid regulations to change the scope or volume of covered services, if they so desired. To encourage participation, Medicare was designed the first payer for services covered by both. It was noted that the states would probably pay a higher amount to the individual clinics under a Medicaid waiver, but it was postulated that "the savings resulting from these projects should more than offset these costs. This saving should accrue from the reduction in utilization of inpatient services...and emergency room services." [10]

A contract was awarded by HCFA to the Center for Health Administration Studies (CHAS) at the University of Chicago to evaluate the impact of the MHSP and the Medicare and Medicaid waivers on utilization of municipal health resources in the five participating cities. Among the issues to be addressed by the CHAS evaluation were:

- changes in patients' patterns of use from the public hospital to the neighborhood clinics and the implications for the cost of care for large inner-city populations;
- changes in factors affecting access to medical care in the study communities;
- changes in patterns of health services use by residents of communities near the center; and
- impact on patterns of care among groups with special health care needs, such as the elderly, the chronically ill, and mothers and children. [11]

The Medicare waiver, implemented centrally and uniformly, became operational in each city as soon as the financial officers of the MHSP could set in place the necessary billing and financial reporting mechanisms. These administrative requirements presented stumbling blocks to the programs, only two of which were able to bill under the Medicare waiver by the end of the first program year. However, during the next year use of the Medicare waiver increased significantly. Specific clinics in Baltimore, Milwaukee, and San Jose were found to have attracted large numbers of Medicare beneficiaries, particularly by the dental services. Cincinnati deemphasized the Medicare waiver in order to avoid competing with private physicians, and Medicare utilization in Cincinnati remained disproportionately low.

Across all five cities, from FY 1980, the first year during which the waiver program received substantial utilization, waiver reimbursement approximately doubled each successive fiscal year through the end of 1982 (see Table 2.1). Total reimbursement for all cities rose from $45,130 in FY 1979 to $1,298,550 in FY 1980, $2,667,810 in FY 1981, and $5,225,000 in FY 1982. San Jose and Baltimore had the highest reimbursements under the Medicare waiver for a cumulative total by December 1982 of $3,034,000

Table 3.1   MHSP Medicare Waivers HCFA Total[1] Reimbursement through December 1982 (in thousands)

| City | Fiscal year | | | | Cumulative total |
	1979	1980	1981	1982	
Baltimore	NA	$98	$517	$2,400	$3,015
Cincinnati	$8	32	65	180	285
San Jose	NA	500	1,164	1,370	3,034
St. Louis	NA	156	419	444	1,019
Milwaukee	4	513	512	831	1,893
FY totals	45	1,299	2,670	5,225	
Cumulative total all cities through 12/82					$9,246

Notes: Figures have been rounded.

    [1] Total = Reimbursements for Routine and Ancillary Services

Source: Health Care Financing Administration, Office of Demonstrations and Evaluations, Department of Health and Human Services, unpublished data, 1983.

and $3,015,000, respectively, compared to only $285,000 in Cincinnati. Milwaukee and St. Louis were in the middle of the range with cumulative reimbursements of $1,893,000 and $1,019,000, respectively. During FY 1981, San Jose's Medicare waiver reimbursement was more than double that of the next highest city. During FY 1982, reimbursement under the Medicare waiver in Baltimore more than quadrupled from the previous year and was almost double that of San Jose. During 1982 growth was dramatic in Baltimore and quite rapid in absolute terms in San Jose and Milwaukee as well.[12] The heavy use of special services such as dentistry and vision care by nonpoor and nonminority elderly raised questions of distributional equity for the program staff in San Jose. In Baltimore and other cities, program staff were most concerned about the fiscal impact of a discontinuation of the waiver once the demonstration period ended.

At the federal level, the Medicaid waiver could only be authorized. Each city had to develop a waiver proposal, submit an application to its state Medicaid agency, and lobby for approval. The states were slow to respond, and only four states expressed a willingness to participate. Ohio declined to participate on the grounds that state law already provided for clinic payment on the same basis as hospital outpatient departments. The California and Missouri waiver applications requested only a change to cost-based reimbursement, while Maryland and Wisconsin added preventive and outreach services not otherwise covered. These waiver requests were submitted by the states to HCFA during mid-1980. However, the states generally experienced rapidly increasing Medicaid expenditures during this period and were instituting administrative, eligibility, and service changes to reduce the growth in costs, so attention was diverted from the waivers. The cities were having difficulties in setting up acceptable billing mechanisms as well; therefore there were delays in the actual commencement of billing under the Medicaid waivers. St. Louis and Baltimore began to bill in 1981, and Baltimore negotiated a modified agreement for increased rates (though not cost based) in 1982, but neither Milwaukee nor San Jose billed under the Medicaid waivers until late 1982. Only Baltimore had received claimed costs or payments under the Medicaid waiver by FY 1981. By the end of June 1983, the cities reportedly had received total reimbursements of $1,099,400, ranging from $0 in Milwaukee to $507,800 in San Jose (see Table 2.2).[13] The Medicaid waiver thus did not bring significant financial resources into the program until late in the course of the demonstration.

The Medicare waiver represented a major improvement in the environment for the MHSP clinics in that it evoked substantial increases in utilization at many sites and paid a very favorable rate for services. St. Louis, however, experienced difficulty in financing production of the more costly services (dentures, eyeglasses) despite the cost-based reimbursement. Should the waivers terminate as planned at the end of the demonstration, the clinics will face a much more constricted reimbursement environment.

Table 3.2   MHSP Medicaid Waivers HCFA Total Reimbursement
through June 1983

City	Cumulative number of visits	Total HCFA reimbursement
Baltimore (2/81)	17,600[1]	$131,400
San Jose[2] (10/81)	9,300[2]	507,800[2]
St. Louis (6/81)	25,000	461,000
Milwaukee (9/83)	(40)	(800)
Total		$1,099,400
		—From States' Quarterly Reports and from HCFA's ODR for CA.

Notes: [1] Partially reported

[2] Excludes Clinic S. Reflects only interim payments.

Date = Date city began implementing the waiver. Reimbursement is retroactive for all cities to 2/81 and will continue through 12/84.

Source: Health Care Financing Administration, Office of Demonstrations and Evaluations, Department of Health and Human Services, unpublished data, 1983.

The impact of the waivers on utilization patterns and total costs per person will not be known until the findings of the CHAS evaluation are reported in 1985.

States were generally reluctant and slow to approve the Medicaid waivers, each of which had the apparent short-term prospect of raising state costs by covering more services or paying the clinics more for a visit. Medicaid budget increases were of major concern to policymakers in all the states involved and only intensified during the course of the MHSP. By the final year of the program, the Medicaid waivers were tentatively in place in all four states. Although the effects of these waivers theoretically could have been substantial, given the large Medicaid patient load at most of the clinics and the advantage of cost-based reimbursement over the previous low Medicaid fee schedules, the clinics were not able to capitalize on the potential until late in the program. By 1981 and 1982, some states were discussing capitated prepayment and preferred provider contracts for Medicaid patients as alternatives to the waiver (St. Louis and San Jose).

Transfer of Resources

SOURCES OF STAFF

Among the original MHSP goals was the expectation that staffing resources would shift from the public hospitals to neighborhood-based MHSP clinics. This goal was in keeping with the principal objective of shifting primary care patients out of the emergency room and outpatient department and into a less costly neighborhood clinic. In general, except in Milwaukee, the anticipated transfer of staff from the public hospital to MHSP clinics did not occur; rather, new personnel were recruited or health department personnel were transferred. The patterns varied city by city and clinic by clinic, as well as by type of personnel.

Some patterns were consistent across cities. The MHSP clinics which had previously operated as traditional public health clinics continued to use public health nursing and support personnel as carryover staffing. In Cincinnati and St. Louis most clinic sites fit this pattern, although each city integrated one preexisting comprehensive community health center into its MHSP. Expansions in physician, nursing, technical, and other support staff were effected by recruiting through the health department structure. Both Cincinnati and St. Louis closed some health department clinics (MHSP and other sites) during the course of the project, and some staff were shifted from the defunct clinics into the remaining sites. When Milwaukee's county hospital-operated Center J was closed and the county withdrew its staff from Center L, the personnel were transferred back to the county hospital where they had originated. St. Louis was another city which had an opportunity to shift hospital staff into the neighborhood clinics due to the city decision to close Homer G. Phillips hospital. Yet this situation did not result in any systematic movement of personnel for several reasons: the hospital closure provoked an extremely angry reaction from black citizens and workers who perceived transfer proposals as threatening the possibility of reopening the inpatient facility; since outpatient and emergency services at the facility remained in operation, only inpatient personnel were displaced, mainly to other city inpatient institutions; and the historic division between hospital and health department activities militated against the possibility of easy mingling of staff.

Baltimore brought one existing public health clinic and a satellite into the MHSP. These two clinics at first kept their small contingent of public health nursing and support staff but added all new provider, technical, and administrative personnel. The physicians at these and all of Baltimore's sites were originally affiliated with Baltimore City Hospitals because they were members of Chesapeake Physicians Professional Association (CPPA), the group of M.D.'s which provided staff under contract to both the hospital and to the MHSP. It is not accurate, however, to describe the doctors as having been shifted from the hospital. The individuals were generally new recruits hired to staff MHSP and other CPPA ambulatory care operations and were given admitting privileges at the hospital. Physician assistants and nurse-midwives were also recruited and employed by the physician group. When the CPPA group was replaced in 1980 by the Central Maryland Medical Group (CMMG), another multispecialty private group practice, this group became the employer of all physicians and mid-level practitioners for the MHSP clinics. A third physician group of family practitioners affiliated with the University of Maryland later signed a contract to staff a fifth clinic. Dentistry, ophthalmology, optometry, and podiatry were all provided in the MHSP clinics under contract by private groups of specialists who recruit and hire their own staff. The city health department hires the nursing, clerical, and other support staff in the clinics staffed by CMMG, and Bon Secours Hospital, which is the backup facility for the clinic staffed by the family practice group, hires the nursing staff for this site but receives funds for salaries from the health department. The only direct staffing contribution from the public hospital to the MHSP was a part-time social worker and one laboratory technician paid by the hospital.

Milwaukee, by virtue of its unusual program structure, experienced more public hospital involvement in MHSP staffing than any other city, at least at the outset of the program. The contribution may be described as a shift to the neighborhood clinics. The Milwaukee design incorporated as an MHSP site a large ambulatory care clinic already operated by the county hospital at a downtown inner-city location. It also established two new public clinics, the primary care component of which was provided entirely under county hospital auspices through the county budget. The physician, nursing, and other support staff for primary care services were all hired by the hospital administration in collaboration with the affiliated medical college. The new clinic operations were staffed mainly by transfer of hospital personnel. The county in 1981 closed the large downtown clinic facility, which predated the MHSP, in an effort to reduce budget deficits at the hospital complex. This clinic closure was a function of the peculiar political structure of Milwaukee's project. The rationale was that the proportional tax levy contribution was much higher at the downtown clinic than in the outpatient department of the hospital. The staff displaced by the clinic closing then shifted not to the smaller remaining clinics but to the hospital. County staffing was unilaterally terminated by the city health department at one of the smaller clinics subsequent to the county-initiated closing of the large site and these personnel also returned to the county hospital. By the end of the demonstration period, only a limited primary care staff was provided at one MHSP clinic site by the county hospital. Staffing of preventive services remained under health department control throughout the project, while independent providers of a variety of additional services recruited and hired their own employees with no hospital or health department involvement.

San Jose's project design, while placing the county hospital director in the MHSP project director's role, did not really allow for shifts of staff from the hospital to the clinic sites. The MHSP clinics were operated by existing community health centers under subcontract, and these private, nonprofit, independent organizations did all their own recruiting and hiring of staff—from physicians to van drivers. Even the inclusion, late in the project, of a former county public health department clinic as an MHSP site resulted in only minimal hospital staff transfer: an administrator from the hospital temporarily became part-time clinic manager to recruit additional physician and support staff, who were hired from outside the hospital.

In summary, staff were generally not shifted from the public hospital to the MHSP clinics, as had been anticipated, except in Milwaukee. There were several reasons for this. The grant funding and responsibility for MHSP implementation were placed in the health department in four of five cities, and historic patterns showed little interaction between the health department and hospital bureaucracies for shared projects. This split was further complicated in Milwaukee and San Jose because the public hospital was a county facility while the MHSP grant went to the city. Personnel operations are particularly difficult to share. With no dollars coming to the hospital, the likelihood of its giving up positions was low. The fact that so many clinics had historically operated as public health clinics was discouraging to hospital involvement, especially in St. Louis and Cincinnati. Those clinics which previously operated as independent community health centers were equally likely to maintain independent hiring patterns. No clear mechanism existed in most of the cities for transferring personnel from the hospital to clinics operating under different auspices. Finally, in the environment of budgetary constraint felt in all five cities, the local public officials did not take dollars or personnel out of the public hospital a move them to the MHSP clinics. While hospital budgets were scrutinized and sometimes cut, at no point did leaders articulate a policy of shifting resources from the hospital to the clinics, and in fact clinics were closed and their budgets were cut as well.

HEALTH BUDGET ALLOCATIONS DURING THE MHSP

Another approach to assessing the degree to which resources may have been transferred from the public hospital to the neighborhood-based clinics is to examine how localities reallocated funds to alternative health programs over the course of the demonstration. The health and hospitals budgets of the five cities were buffeted by an economic recession, state and local tax limitation measures, loss of federal revenues, and health care cost inflation.

Between fiscal years 1978 and 1982, Baltimore's municipal operating budget rose by 19.6 percent, and the share of the budget claimed by health and hospitals rose from 7 to 9 percent of the total. During this period non-municipal revenues to both health and hospitals rose dramatically, allowing the city subsidy to drop substantially. The Baltimore health department's expenditures rose from $35.3 million in FY 1978 to $47.3 million in 1982, primarily due to an increase in state mental health funds, while its proportion of the city operating budget went up to 4.4 percent from 3.7 percent. At the same time Baltimore City Hospitals' budget grew from $37.9 million to $59.6 million, or from 3.3 to 4.6 percent of total city operating costs. However, the city tax levy contribution to the health department dropped from $8.7 million to under $6 million, and city tax levy going to the public hospital plummeted from $5 million in 1978 to under $1.2 million in 1982, because of nearly doubled patient care revenues at the hospital and aggressive grantsmanship by the health department.

The Cincinnati health department's budget grew by 52 percent from FY 1977 to FY 1981, or from $14.7 million to $22.5 million. The local contribution increased by 72 percent during this period, going from a low of 36 percent of the budget in 1978 to 44 percent in 1981. It is likely to have increased even more in the two subsequent years. The city budget increased by 23 percent between 1979 (the earliest available data) and 1981. In 1979, the health department accounted for 17 percent of city expenditures, falling to 15 percent in 1981. The budget of the Cincinnati General Hospital, a state rather than a local expense, increased from $60.6 million in FY 1977 to $92.6 million in FY 1981, or 53 percent. The hospital received a substantial local tax levy contribution, not from Cincinnati but from Hamilton County, a subsidy which grew by 49 percent from $9.2 million to $13.6 million in this period, maintaining a share of approximately 15 percent of the hospital's revenues.

The City of Milwaukee operates the municipal health department. The county of Milwaukee is responsible for public hospital services. Milwaukee's city health department had a 1978 budget of $11.1 million, or 5 percent of the city budget. Although the health department budget dropped in 1979, it rose to $13.8 million by 1981. From FY 1978 to FY 1981, the city budget grew by 26 percent, the municipal health department budget grew by 24 percent, and health department expenditures maintained about a 5 percent share of the city budget. During this period, the health department was able to increase nonlocal resources from just over $2 million, or 20 percent of its budget, to almost $3.5 million, or 25 percent, although city expenditures also rose modestly in absolute terms. The city general fund contributed 77 percent of the health department budget in 1978 and 72 percent in 1981. The MHSP contributed only a small amount to this new nonlocal revenue since patient care revenue went to independent providers. Community Development Block Grant funds represented the largest increment.

The Milwaukee County Medical Complex, which included the county general hospital, the rehabilitation and chronic hospital, the mental health center, and the downtown ambulatory care facility, accounted for 19 percent of the county's expenditures in FY 1978. Milwaukee County General Hospital alone had 1978 expenditures of $61.5 million, or 11 percent of the county budget; general hospital costs increased to $78.3 million in 1981, 14.4 percent of county expenditures. By FY 1981, despite removal of the chronic hospital from the county budget, general hospital and health center (three MHSP sites) expenditures constituted 27 percent of all county outlays. Costs at the general hospital increased by 32 percent, while health center costs doubled. Although two sites were added, the budget for preexisting Clinic J rose by $75,000, a sum equal to the combined costs of the two other centers; this was a major reason why county officials decided to close the facility at the end of 1981. At the general hospital, combined costs of the outpatient department and the emergency room increased by 64 percent between FY 1978 and FY 1981. County funds subsidized the general hospital by about $7 million in 1978 and $8 million in 1981.

The St. Louis municipal budget grew by 27 percent between FY 1978 and FY 1981. In 1981, St. Louis expended $11 million, or 3 percent, of the city budget on its health division. This amount represented an increase of 48 percent over the 1978 figure of $7.4 million, or 2.6 percent of the city budget. The local government contribution had increased from 47 percent to 51 percent, and had grown from $3.5 million to $5.6 million. The costs of public (two acute, one chronic, and one rehabilitation) hospitals in St. Louis grew from $64.1 million in 1978 to $72.9 million in 1981, or by only 14 percent. The deceleration in hospital expenditures was achieved at the cost of closing one of the two municipal general hospitals. These costs represented 22.5 percent of the city budget in 1978 and 20.2 percent in 1981. The presence of the MHSP exerted a protective influence on the health division's budget, particularly after FY 1980 when the growth in state and federal revenues began to slow and the city substantially increased its support for health division operations.

Although the Santa Clara County health department has no direct role in the MHSP, it does provide a range of preventive primary care services, especially through its health administration/public health division. The department also operates mental health, public guardian, drug abuse, alcohol, and emergency medical services programs. Santa Clara County devoted $36.9 million to its health department in FY 1978. This figure grew rapidly by 44 percent to $53.3 million in FY 1981. However, the health department budget dropped by 8 percent to $48.8 million for FY 1982, reflecting local property tax cuts and the California state budget crisis as well as federal categorical program cuts. The public health division lost 21 percent of its resources and 24 percent of its funded positions during this period when the impact of Proposition 13 became severe. Data for other county expenditures, including the budget of the county hospital, were not available. It was projected that the loss of resources for services to the elderly, maternal and child health, and well-baby clinics would lead to more patient visits at the public hospital and the community clinics, including the MHSP sites.

Summary

It is very difficult to draw any inferences about the impact of the MHSP on hospital and health department budget allocations. It is likely that the impact was minimal on hospital resource allocation in all the cities. The MHSP may have exerted a protective influence on health department budgets in Baltimore, Cincinnati, and St. Louis, but only in the areas of direct personal health services. In Milwaukee, the health department may have been able to preserve its preventive services with MHSP funds. Santa Clara County's health functions appear to have been unaffected. No pattern of redirection of hospital resources to neighborhood-based care has been detected in any city as a specific result of the MHSP.

Notes

1. Patricia Maloney Alt, "Field Associate Final Report for Columbia University, Conservation of Human Resources: Municipal Health Services Program Evaluation."
2. Schramm and Christopherson, 10.
3. Ibid.
4. Ibid.
5. Ibid.
6. Ibid.
7. Center for Health Administration Studies, *Evaluation of MHSP Phase II Report* (Graduate School of Business, University of Chicago, January 31, 1983).
8. "A Review of the Billing, Accounts Receivable, Patient Mix, Service Mix and Related Management Reporting Systems of Five Selected Health Centers in the Municipal Health Services Program," Report prepared by Laventhol and Horwath, Certified Public Accountants, New York, New York, November 1982.
9. Acting Assistant Administrator for Demonstrations and Evaluations, Department of Health, Education, and Welfare, "Memorandum on Municipal Health Services Program" (Health Care Financing Administration, May 17, 1978).
10. Ibid.
11. Judy Lippman, Office of Demonstrations and Evaluations, Department of Health, Education, and Welfare, "Memorandum to Clifton R. Gaus on Status of Robert Wood Johnson Foundation Municipal Health Services Program (MHSP) and HCFA Involvement in the MHSP" (Health Care Financing Administration, September 8, 1978).
12. Health Care Financing Administration, Office of Demonstrations and Evaluations, unpublished reports to the Municipal Health Services Program National Advisory Board, 1982 and 1983.
13. Ibid.

4

The Impact of National Environmental Influences

The Municipal Health Services Program (MHSP) was implemented in the context of a rapidly changing national environment. A number of general parameters—political, economic, demographic, and social—and several others specific to the health services arena, were critical to the program's success. Their influence upon the course of the program was pervasive, both facilitating and impeding implementation. These environmental influences include trends in the economy, employment levels, and public resources; federal and state policies (especially health services policy); changes in the supply and use of health resources (particularly physicians and hospitals); the relative positions of public sector, private nonprofit, and proprietary institutions; and the general willingness of society to devote resources to health care.

This chapter will discuss the importance of state and national developments for the implementation of a local health services initiative. State and federal health policy changes are among the most critical influences upon programs at the local level. The contracting economy, which in most of the demonstration cities followed national trends, created unanticipated constraints and burdens. Trends in the supply of physicians and hospital beds, reflected in intensified competition in the local health system, affected the structure and utilization of the demonstration projects. It is fair to say that these forces had important, perhaps critical, effects upon the implementation and operation of the Municipal Health Services Program.

Implicit Assumptions

It is also fair to say that the perceptions of the Robert Wood Johnson Foundation, in consultation with its collaborators, about the environment for inner-city health services were responsible for the initiation of the program in the mid-1970s and were implicit in the MHSP design. Perhaps most important was the assumption that private physician services were and would remain unavailable to inner-city populations. Similarly, it was assumed that municipal hospital outpatient departments (OPDs) and emergency rooms (ERs) represented the primary alternative to private physician services for these populations. Both assumptions were in agreement with the conventional analysis of urban health care delivery in the mid-1970s.[1] The baseline survey of health care utilization by residents of selected target neighborhoods in the demonstration cities by the University of Chicago Center for Health Administration Studies (CHAS) disclosed, however, that a majority of residents in these neighborhoods reported private physicians as their usual source of care and, except for St. Louis, only a small minority reported dependence upon the public hospital. The potential for shifting utilization from the public hospital to the neighborhood clinics was substantially lessened by this reality.[2] The CHAS findings became available in 1981, and supported evidence suggested by the slow buildup of visit volume and anecdotal reports early during program implementation of alternative sources of care.

The Foundation's initial design implicitly assumed a local environment in which the municipality exercised responsibility for and control over public health and public hospital services. The issue of a local government structure with responsibility for health care was critical to successful implementation of the MHSP. Nevertheless, the selection of grantees necessitated a compromise in the model, for in only two cities did the municipality operate both the hospital and the health department, and in one city, it operated neither. A broader definition of local government was needed, and was, in fact, accepted, but the mayor remained the political leader upon whom the program focussed.

Although the shift in the nation's health policy agenda from expanding access to containing costs had begun in the mid-1970s (and this is reflected in the dual goals of the MHSP to increase access to high-quality preventive and therapeutic services while reducing costs), it was assumed at the outset that the basic mechanisms for financing publicly sponsored health care would remain intact and that improved service organization and financial practices would allow localities to better their revenues from Medicaid, Medicare, and private payers. The Johnson Foundation correctly anticipated that responsibility for service delivery would be shifted increasingly from the federal government to the state and local levels, but program administrators assumed as late as 1979 that state and local budgets would be strengthened relative to the federal budget and that unprecedentedly large surpluses would accrue at the state and local levels leading to an expanded role as initiators and sponsors of new programs.[3] The national economic recession, however, caused a rapid drop in state tax revenues, producing intense pressure on Medicaid budgets, and cutbacks in health and other programs. Urban localities generally experienced budget cutbacks by the turn of the decade as well. These issues will be discussed at greater length below.

One final assumption central to the Johnson Foundation's decision to launch the MHSP was the vital importance of maintaining the viability of the cities' public general hospitals, a conclusion inferred from the findings of the Commission on Public General Hospitals, which the Foundation had supported from 1976 to 1978. The MHSP was specifically intended to carry out the commission's recommendation that public hospitals should become broad-based community resources, in part through "planning and arranging for neighborhood-based primary care services for community residents who do not have access to such care."[4] The future of the public hospital was the overriding issue when the MHSP was conceived. However, in only two of the cities was the public hospital a major participant in the MHSP; its role was that of a service provider in one and that of a limited negotiator, rather than leader, in the other. The public hospital had not adopted the agenda of the commission or of the Foundation. In fact, four of the localities participating in the MHSP considered discontinuing operation of their public hospitals and two cities took steps to close or spin off their facilities. The MHSP functioned from the beginning essentially as a health department program in four of the five cities; the proposals that received awards were submitted by health departments with hospital acquiescence. In St. Louis, the MHSP proposal originated in the office of the director of health and hospitals and was developed by physicians from the hospital division, but the funded project was placed in the health division for administration.

Understanding the implicit assumptions at the outset of the program provides a background for mapping shifts in perceptions and in goals, the sources of compromises and adaptations, and the overt influences of the environment on the choices that were made by local program administrators, local political leaders, the central program managers, and the Johnson Foundation.

The Economic and Political Environment

The Municipal Health Services Program was launched during a period of reasonable growth in the economy. After the recession of 1974–75, the gross national product (GNP) grew in 1976–78 at an annual rate of about 5.5 percent (in constant 1972 dollars).[5] Growth, however, slackened, and the nation entered a recession in 1980. A brief recovery was followed by a new recession beginning in July 1981, with a 2.6 percent drop in real GNP by early 1982. The recession was the worst since the Depression and persisted into 1983. In early 1983, less than 68 percent of manufacturing capacity was in operation, and the national unemployment rate reached almost 11 percent, also a postwar record. The recession hit hardest at cities dependent on manufacturing, and its impact was variable across the five MHSP cities. Baltimore, Milwaukee, and Cincinnati experienced higher unemployment rates than St. Louis or San Jose (see Table 3.1).[6]

The loss of health insurance benefits by unemployed workers rapidly gained prominence as a national health policy issue. By the end of 1982, the Congressional Budget Office estimated that nationally 10.7 million workers and dependents had lost health coverage as a result of layoffs.[7] A more conservative estimate by the Robert Wood Johnson Foundation, which took into account extended benefits and working spouses' coverage, concluded that from 5.5 to 7 million persons lacked insurance due to job loss.[8] At the local level, health services managers for the MHSP sites anticipated during 1981 that clinic utilization would be boosted by unemployed workers who could no longer afford private sector health care. St. Louis, Baltimore, and Cincinnati reported some enrollment in the MHSP system of the newly unemployed. Public hospitals began to see an increase in utilization result-

Table 4.1   Unemployment Rates for Cities Participating in the MHSP

Location	Annual rates			Month and year of peak	Rate at peak
	1980	1981	1982		
Baltimore					
City	9.2%	10.3%	11.4%	Jan. '82	12.1%
Baltimore County	7.8%	8.2%	10.2%	Jan. '82	10.6%
Cincinnati					
City	N.A.	N.A.	13.2%	Jan. '83	15.3%
Hamilton County	6.7%	8.6%	10.2%	Jan. '83	11.9%
Milwaukee					
City	N.A.	13.1%	13.1%	Jan. '83	15.8%
Milwaukee County	6.3%	11.0%	11.0%	Jan. '83	13.2%
St. Louis					
City	8.6%	9.5%	10.8%	Feb. '83	12.2%
St. Louis County	6.4%	6.7%	7.8%	Feb. '83	9.3%
San Jose					
City	N.A.	N.A.	N.A.	N.A.	N.A.
Santa Clara County	5.1%	5.9%	7.5%	Jan. '83	9.1%

Source: Division of Research and Analysis, Maryland Department of Human Resources; Division of Research and Statistics, Ohio Bureau of Employment Services; Bureau of Research and Statistics, Wisconsin Department of Industry, Labor and Human Relations; Division of Employment Security, Missouri Department of Labor and Industrial Relations; and Employment Data and Research Division, California Employment Development Department.

ing from cuts in Medicaid eligibility and payment schedules in some states, as well as the loss of private health insurance, reversing a long-term decline in utilization.

The recession had a direct effect upon states and localities as well as the federal government by virtue of declines in the growth of tax revenues. The states, which depend heavily upon sales and income taxes that are sensitive to fluctuations in the economy, were particularly vulnerable. The states had adopted these elastic taxes during a relatively protracted period of economic expansion and had built up surpluses during the 1970s.[9] In a number of states, these surpluses prompted tax revolts, leading in the early 1980s to enactment of a variety of tax limitations in many jurisdictions, including California and Missouri. The economic contracting was reflected in decelerating tax revenues in 1978–82. Nationwide, state tax revenues rose 8.6 percent in FY 1982, compared to 9.3 percent in FY 1981, without adjusting for inflation. Concomitantly, demands upon state and local government for services increased because of the recession. Per capita spending by state and local government, however, began to decrease in 1979 from a peak of $887 in 1978 to $839 in 1982.[10] The turning point in the rate of growth of federal aid to states and localities was also reached in 1978; until then it had been the fastest-growing component of state and local revenues. Federal aid declined from $231 per capita in 1978 to $174 in 1982. Fiscal year 1982 marked the first absolute decline in the volume of federal aid to state and local government in 27 years; from $94.8 billion in 1981 the amount dropped to $88.8 billion, or 6.3 percent.[11] The combined effects of declining federal aid (proportionally, then absolutely), the recession, and the tax revolt led to serious state budget problems.

The states almost universally are constrained by their constitutions to operate with balanced budgets. During fiscal years 1981 and 1982 most states had to scramble to avoid deficits. An August 1982 report found that 40 states had initiated some kind of tax increase in 1981 or 1982.[12] In February 1983, the *New York Times* reported that in FY 1982, 22 states projected deficits; 15 states had surpluses; 13 expected to break even; 33 had raised or were raising taxes; 38 had cut their budgets, frozen hiring, laid off workers, deferred payments, speeded up collections, transferred money from trust funds, or resorted to other fiscal restraints.[13] A survey of the budget condition of 41 states conducted by the National Governor's Association in January 1983 revealed that of the five states in which MHSP cities are located, two reported deficits (California $1,651 million and Wisconsin $266 million), two reported a break-even position (Ohio and Maryland), and Missouri projected a surplus of $63 million.[14] Missouri's Republican governor has consistently relied upon optimistic estimates of revenue since 1981 to avoid asking the Democratic legislature or the voters to approve tax increases. In fact, Missouri has had to struggle to remain in the break-even category. All five states had raised taxes (generally excise taxes) and used various means to cut expenditures. Ohio had raised its income tax and Wisconsin its sales tax, unequivocal signs of fiscal hardship since both are especially unpopular taxes to increase. Missouri voters, through the initiative process, increased the sales tax to meet teachers' salaries, but the new revenue was to be partially offset by a property tax rollback.[15]

Through 1982, among the fastest rising components of state expenditures was the Medicaid program. From 1978 to 1979, Medicaid costs rose annually 17.9 percent while state operating budgets increased only 9.3 percent.[16] In FY 1981 Medicaid outlays grew 23 percent, but in 1982 the rate of increase was held to 10 percent. The states had exercised whatever administrative flexibility they could muster to reduce payments to providers and to tighten certification and reimbursement procedures. Until 1981 most states had avoided eligibility reduction or elimination of services, and had instead limited the volume of services provided as a means of saving money. While state budget crises of late 1981 and early 1982 led to more drastic measures, concurrent congressional action authorized the states to experiment with a number of alternatives. Although earlier options were unable to affect the inflationary dynamics of the medical care system, many of the new approaches directly address its organizational and cost elements. Further, federal eligibility cuts in the Aid to Families with Dependent Children (AFDC) program have meant that persons bumped from AFDC have also lost Medicaid eligibility.

Among the changes authorized by Congress was the offer of waivers of federal regulations to allow reimbursement for home- and community-based services as an alternative to nursing home care, the largest component of Medicaid expenditure in most states. By mid-1982, 29 states had filed 38 waiver applications under this authority. A second major change authorized states to apply for waivers of the freedom of choice provision which allowed beneficiaries unrestricted choice of physicians and provider institutions, leading, according to critics, to overuse of these services at unreasonably high rates. The new flexibility permits states not only to "lock in" high users to designated providers but to contract with selected hospitals, to enroll recipients for care in cost-effective health maintenance organizations, or to require preauthorization of all services by physician case managers. By July 1982, 28 applications for waiver of freedom of choice were received by the Health Care Financing Administration. A third major legislative change authorized the states to develop alternatives to cost-based hospital and nursing home reimbursement, for which only a few states had obtained waivers previously. States by July 1982 had submitted 99 applications to alter their systems of payment to nursing homes and 20 to reform hospital reimbursement. By September 1982, five states, including Missouri, had adopted prospective hospital payment plans. Maryland was one of the few states which had an approved state hospital rate-setting plan prior to the new legislation.[17]

California responded to the new flexibility with the most far-reaching changes in its Medi-Cal program. Legislation enacted in July 1982 authorized selective hospital provider contracts to cover services to Medi-Cal beneficiaries. The law also allows private insurers to negotiate selective contracts with hospitals for service provision and instructs the state to enter into Medi-Cal contracts with physicians for their services to beneficiaries beginning in July 1983. The law designated a single special state representative, known as the "Medi-Cal czar," to negotiate Medi-Cal contracts with California hospitals under a competitive bidding process. His powers were to last for one year, at the end of which he would become an employee of the new California Medical Assistance Commission which would assume responsibility for contract negotiations. The state of California was trying to avoid a looming budget deficit by cutting at least $300 million from its $5 billion Medi-Cal and medically indigent program. The competitive bidding was to save $100 million, while eligibility and benefit cuts were to produce the balance of the savings. California's plan to contract with cost-effective providers was approved by the federal government under a waiver of the freedom of choice rule in September 1982.[18] The selective provider contracting program began to solicit hospital bids in the fall of 1982 and the first hospitals began accepting Medi-Cal patients under the new contracts on February 1, 1983. The competitive bidding process eliminated from Medi-Cal participation some hospitals which had previously carried heavy Medi-Cal patient loads. For example, in the San Francisco area, where nine of 15 competing hospitals won contracts, one hospital which had cared for 26 percent of the area's Medi-Cal patients failed to be awarded a contract.[19] The state Medi-Cal negotiator describes California's policy as a shift to a price-driven, economic system from the previous socially determined system of payment for health services. He contrasts this to the choice by other states of a regulatory approach following a public utility or rate-setting model (New York, Massachusetts, Maryland, and Connecticut).[20] Although the new California contracts generally use the traditional per diem dollar amount as the unit for pricing, there has been a radical philosophical change. The potential exists for dramatic shifts in patient utilization patterns and particularly in physician/hospital relationships. Pricing patterns set under Medi-Cal may have a strong influence on how other payers approach hospitals under new preferred provider organization (PPO) arrangements as well as the acceptability of hospital charges. Given the generally low level of occupancy in California hospitals, the newly heated competition may lead to some institutional failures, and mergers of others. California's experience will be watched closely by the rest of the country as state legislatures continue to deal with containing Medicaid costs. It is among the most radical of the many new approaches to holding down or reversing the growth in health care costs.

The federal role in changing health policy has been mentioned in the previous discussion of changing state health policy during the course of the Municipal Health Services Program and should be reviewed briefly. The issue of cost containment first gained a prominent position on the federal health policy agenda during the Carter administration, which made a futile effort to enact legislation setting a hospital cost cap. With the election of Ronald Reagan the policy agenda changed dramatically. While cost containment gained further prominence, the approach proposed was antiregulatory. The Reagan administration enunciated a number of specific priorities in health policy, most of which exemplified the administration's general approach to domestic policy. The most pervasive influence was the philosophy that the size of the federal government must be reduced, domestic spending cut, and defense spending increased. The specific health policy initiatives all derive from these administration imperatives.

First, the Reagan administration attempted to reduce the rate of growth of spending for both entitlement programs and discretionary domestic programs. In health, the Medicaid program's federal budget contribution was limited to an annual rise of under 5 percent from 1982 through 1984. At the same time, eligibility for the program was tightened through reductions in the AFDC program. Medicaid grants to the states totalled $17.4 billion in 1982, an increase of 3.4 percent from $16.8 billion in 1981. Categorical health programs sustained cuts approximating 15 percent between 1981 and 1982, while Medicare remained essentially unscathed, although beneficiary contributions in the form of premiums, coinsurance, and deductibles were increased. The prospects are for Medicare to absorb a greater proportion of future cuts because its costs are increasing more rapidly than those of Medicaid following the recent changes in that program and congressional leaders believe that the "safety net" for the poor must be protected.[21]

A major theme of the Reagan administration has been the devolution of responsibility for social programs from the federal government to the states. In the health arena, this objective has been pursued through grouping categorical programs into block grants. Although Congress did not approve the full extent of the administration's proposals for collapsing categorical programs into blocks, between 1981 and 1982 four major health block grants were approved covering 25 previous categorical programs in the areas of maternal and child health, mental health and drug and alcohol abuse, preventive health services, and primary care. Most states began operating the first three block grants during 1982 with a budget reduction of about 15 percent from the previous year's funding level.[22] Implementation of the primary care block grant was delayed to give states more time to develop mechanisms for administering such programs as community health centers, which had originated with direct federal-to-local funding flows. Following the enactment of the first of nine congressionally approved block grants, the administration launched a series of negotiations with representatives of the states over a proposed New Federalism initiative, in which the states were to take over a number of additional programs, notably AFDC, as a trade-off for assumption of the Medicaid program by the federal government. The terms of the exchange could not be agreed upon by the National Governors' Association and the administration, and by early 1983, this New Federalism proposal had died. Seven additional social program block grants were proposed for FY 1983 but were not approved.

Assessment of the impact of the block grants varies. The funding cuts were substantial and states generally did not replace lost federal funds. A report by Professor Richard Nathan of Princeton University's Urban and Regional Research Center indicated that during 1982, three of 14 states surveyed replaced from 15 to 25 percent of lost federal funds, five (including

California) replaced less than 10 percent, two shifted resources to supplement some services but had a net reduction, and four (including Ohio and Missouri) made no effort to replace federal funds but cut entitlements further.[23] The survey found that large cities experienced a notable impact from the cuts, and concluded that in at least some cases fears of urban officials that state legislatures would use their expanded authority over funds to funnel resources away from the cities were justified, although health funds were less likely than others to be diverted. St. Louis appeared to lose resources as rural interests in the state legislature shifted funds to rural counties. Categorical health programs in the city suffered large reductions.[24] California required its counties, including Santa Clara, to take over responsibility for the medically indigent adult population, which had previously been covered under Medi-Cal entirely at state expense, and reduced the level of state support. Cincinnati experienced reductions in categorical/block grant funds which the city partially replaced because of strong local support for the health department; this situation was unusual among the MHSP cities. Baltimore generally maintained its position as a major focus for Maryland's public health and Medicaid dollars, since it continued to have a higher proportion of Maryland's poor population and Medicaid beneficiaries than any other locality. Milwaukee experienced funding reductions and increased taxes to maintain its effort in service delivery.

Among the federal policy initiatives favored by the Reagan administration has been the attempt to effect a shift of responsibility for social programs from the public sector to the private sector. While no legislative agenda was proposed to pursue this philosophy, the president enunciated it repeatedly in public remarks defending his efforts to reduce federal spending. The cuts in federal funding during FY 1982 tended to affect nonprofit social service organizations adversely, since many had received substantial proportions of their resources from federal grants. It was difficult for such charitable institutions to play a significant role in replacing resources lost to public services as the result of reductions in federal support when they too had fewer dollars to allocate.[25]

As the Reagan administration moved toward consideration of federal budgets for FYs 1984 and beyond, the combined impacts of economic recession, tax cuts, increased defense spending, and a continuing rise in expenditures for entitlement programs, particularly Medicare and Social Security, led to projected budget deficits which approached $200 billion annually during the mid-1980s, exceeding all previous levels. The concern aroused by these projections and the rapid rate at which both Social Security and Medicare trust funds were approaching insolvency led to the placement of cost containment at the top of the federal health policy agenda. Many analysts have identified the Medicare program's cost reimbursement mechanism and its emphasis on acute hospital care as key contributors to rapid medical-care cost inflation. This perception led Congress to enact in early 1983, with remarkably little debate, the adoption of a system of prospective payment for hospital services to Medicare beneficiaries based on diagnosis related groups (DRGs). This approach had been used only for two years in one state, and can thus be considered experimental. It was extended to all general acute hospitals as of October 1983, and Congress expects to include physician services under prospective payment within a year or two. While the Reagan administration failed as of 1983 to produce its much-heralded proposal to introduce competition into the health services industry, these and other changes have, in fact, acted to do so, as the California Medi-Cal and private insurance initiatives and prospective pricing for the Medicare program demonstrate.

Trends In Health Resources

Among the forces which have led to increasing competition in the health services environment are the recent rapid increase in the number of physicians, the expanding involvement of proprietary enterprise in health service delivery, and demographic and medical practice trends leading to greater use of out-of-hospital services. The physician supply per 100,000 population in the United States grew from 144 in 1960 to 199 in 1980 and is projected to reach 242 by 1990.[26] Although the MHSP had difficulty in recruiting physician staff in its early days, all five cities reported easy availability of physicians by 1981. The most recent available data indicate that the supply of physicians directly engaged in patient care in the five MHSP cities grew in the 1976–81 period as follows: Baltimore city from 3,182 to 3,469; Cincinnati (Hamilton County) from 1,876 to 2,132; Milwaukee (Milwaukee County) from 1,741 to 2,173; St. Louis city from 2,434 to 2,686; and San Jose (Santa Clara County) from 2,253 to 2,829.[27] At the same time, population was dropping in all cities except San Jose.

Additional physicians may be available to previously underserved populations, particularly if an institutional mechanism exists to recruit and organize them, such as the minority private physicians' group in Milwaukee which became a provider in the MHSP. The public sector may continue to have a role as guarantor for those who cannot pay for services, however, as is the case in the Milwaukee program, where patients without resources will be sent to the county hospital after grant subsidies are exhausted. In Baltimore, competition among physicians' groups has developed sufficiently that the MHSP administration was able to substitute a group offering more favorable contract terms when difficulties arose with the original contract group. The Baltimore community has a large number of health maintenance organizations (HMOs), most of which have affiliated physician groups, and although some are primarily targeted to Medicaid enrollees and others seek mainly business employees, there is a certain degree of competition among the HMOs and physician groups. The local medical society sponsored a study which concluded that the existing physician supply could easily handle a significant increase in work load.[28] Although Santa Clara County and San Jose have not been major centers of such activity, California in general has witnessed the rapid growth of physician-sponsored ambulatory surgery centers and urgent care or walk-in centers, which are in direct competition with hospitals for patients. Both San Jose and St. Louis witnessed, during the course of the MHSP project, the planning or actual implementation of a private group practice by the medical staff of the public hospital.

The increasing number of new doctors is likely to lead to competition among physicians for patients and for practice opportunities. The recent changes in reimbursement methods for medical services (first hospital, next physician) will reinforce existing tensions between physicians and hospitals and generate others. The DRG-based prospective payment for Medicare will require hospitals to hold down production costs of services, e.g., physicians' treatment and service-ordering behavior. Potential for fierce conflict exists. In California, the Medi-Cal selective provider contracting program requires existing medical staffs to admit to the staff of a contract hospital any physician who treats Medi-Cal patients, a situation with possibilities for confrontations among physicians and between hospital and staff.

Hospitals thus will be facing competition from physicians as well as from each other. In many areas, hospitals have experienced falling occupancy rates in recent years, at least through 1979. No clear pattern emerges for trends in admissions or days of care in the nation's 50 largest cities. Nationwide, admissions and days of care in nonfederal short-term hospitals showed a steady increase from 1971 through 1981. In the 50 largest cities, days of care in short-term hospitals grew 6.2 percent, from 73.1 million to 77.7 million from 1971 to 1976, but only 1.5 percent, to 78.8 million, between 1976 and 1981. Individual city trends were contradictory: some growing cities showed declines in days overall or for part of the period; some declining cities showed work-load increases for all or part of the period. In St. Louis, days of care increased until 1978 and then fell. In Baltimore and Milwaukee, days rose through 1976, dipped in 1978, then rose again in 1981. In Cincinnati, days declined after 1976. In San Jose, days of care fell in 1971–76, then rose through 1981. Admissions displayed similarly unstable patterns which did not correspond to patterns of days of care. In each participating city, nearly all hospitals showed higher occupancy in 1981 than in 1978, and generally, bed reductions appeared only in public facilities.[29]

Voluntary hospital administrators have perceived their institutions as coming under increased pressure to compete for patients. In the five MHSP cities, voluntary hospitals perceived either that the MHSP clinics might represent a source of new inpatient referrals or, alternatively, that they might deflect into the public hospital patients who otherwise would use the voluntary facility. In three of five cities (Cincinnati and St. Louis excepted) this perception led voluntary hospitals to press for participation in the MHSP. With approval from the program's central managers, the private sector thus became actively involved in the MHSP via voluntary hospitals as clinic sponsors (Milwaukee) or primary referral sources (Baltimore, San Jose), while in Cincinnati the public hospital turned over responsibility for all inpatient pediatric services to the neighboring voluntary children's hospital.

The five cities participating in the MHSP may be unusual for their exclusion from two other notable trends in the hospital industry. None of the cities as of the end of 1982 had experienced proprietary hospital chain acquisitions or management contracts (except for a short-lived contract between a proprietary chain and the county hospital in San Jose). Not a single proprietary hospital operated in the five cities when the MHSP began. This is particularly noteworthy for San Jose, because of the strong record of proprietary activity in the state of California. The five cities had also demonstrated few mergers or service-sharing arrangements among voluntary hospitals as of early 1983. Although preferred provider organizations are growing elsewhere, these five cities showed little such activity as of early 1983, except for the Medi-Cal contracts in San Jose, which are state mandated. It is difficult to estimate the likelihood of such developments in the near future.

Summary

This chapter has described the major influences exerted upon the local health policy environment by economic, political, and health industry trends operating in the broader context of the states and the nation as a whole. While the MHSP is but a small element in the local health arena, the ability of local leaders and program managers to accomplish its goals has been to some degree determined by forces outside their immediate arena. It is possible that the ability of the health department in Cincinnati to recruit highly trained young physicians is related to the expansion of medical school classes and residency training programs in the academic medical centers of New York State, among others. The shortage of dollars for the Medicaid program in most states has made it difficult for MHSP advocates to secure approval of the proposed Medicaid waivers which would improve the clinics' prospects of financial viability. The combined pressures of competition for insured patients and constraints on hospital reimbursement have led in several cities to requests from voluntary hospitals to participate as back-up hospitals for the MHSP. The far-reaching transfer of federal categorical health programs to block grants with reduced funding has meant that health departments, which relied on categorical money for basic support of all their primary care activities, have had great difficulty in maintaining previous levels of services, particularly in the areas of maternal and child health care. Local budget cuts, a reflection of federal and state funding reductions, has meant diminution of services and hours at many MHSP sites, as well as delayed or deferred renovations or equipment purchases. It is evident, then, that the influence of the national environment has been reflected in concrete and specific ways in the implementation of a local health service initiative.

Notes

1. See Karen Davis and Cathy Schoen, *Health and the War on Poverty: A Ten-Year Appraisal* (Washington, D.C.: The Brookings Institution, 1978); Robert Stevens and Rosemary

Stevens, *Welfare Medicine in America: A Case Study of Medicaid* (New York: The Free Press, 1974); Edith M. Davis, Michael L. Millman, and Associates, *Health Care for the Urban Poor: Directions for Policy* (Totowa, N.J.: Rowman & Allanheld, 1983); Mutya San Agustin, "Primary Care in a Tertiary Care Center," *Annals of the New York Academy of Sciences*, 310 (June 1978): 121; Lu Ann Aday, Ronald Andersen, and Gretchen V. Fleming, *Health Care in the U.S.: Equitable for Whom?* (Beverly Hills and London: Sage Publications, 1980).

2. Center for Health Administration Studies, University of Chicago, "Evaluation of Municipal Health Services Program, Phase I (Baseline) Report, HCFA-500-78-00-97," Chicago, March 15, 1982. (Unpublished.)

3. Andrew Greene and Carl J. Schramm, *Municipal Health Services Program, First Annual Report* (The Robert Wood Johnson Foundation, November 1, 1979).

4. Report of the Commission on Public-General Hospitals, *The Future of the Public-General Hospital: An Agenda for Transition* (Chicago: Hospital Research and Educational Trust, 1978), 23–24.

5. U.S. Department of Commerce, *Statistical Abstract of the United States, 1982–83* (Washington, D.C.: GPO, 1982), 418–421.

6. Division of Research and Analysis, Maryland Department of Human Resources, Baltimore, Maryland; Division of Research and Statistics, Ohio Bureau of Employment Services, Columbus, Ohio; Bureau of Research and Statistics, Wisconsin Department of Industry, Labor and Human Resources, Madison, Wisconsin; Division of Employment Security, Missouri Department of Labor and Industrial Relations, St. Louis, Missouri; and Employment Data and Research Division, California Department of Employment Development, San Jose, California.

7. Alice M. Rivlin, director, Congressional Budget Office, "Health Insurance and the Unemployed," Statement before the Subcommittee on Health and Environment, Committee on Energy and Commerce, U.S. House of Representatives, January 24, 1983.

8. Robert J. Blendon, Drew E. Altman, and Saul M. Kilstein, "Health Insurance for the Unemployed and Uninsured," *National Journal* 15 (May 28, 1983):1146–1149.

9. Rochelle L. Stanfield, "States Find Fiscal Modernization Has Ironic Outcomes—Empty Coffers," *National Journal* 14 (August 7, 1982):1379–1381.

10. Rochelle L. Stanfield, "ACIR Study Shoots Down Popular Spending Myths," *National Journal* 15 (February 26, 1983):462.

11. Robert Pear, "Federal Grants Down in '82, First Drop in 27 Years," *New York Times*, May 11, 1983.

12. Stanfield, "States Find Fiscal Modernization Has Ironic Outcomes—Empty Coffers," 1379–1381.

13. "Many States Facing Need for New Taxes to Balance Budgets," *New York Times*, February 22, 1983.

14. Rochelle L. Stanfield, "Governors, Mayors Turn from Seeking More Power to Fending Off Aid Cuts," *National Journal* 15 (January 22, 1983):166–169.

15. Stanfield, "States Find Fiscal Modernization Has Ironic Outcomes—Empty Coffers."

16. Linda E. Demkovich, "For States Squeezed by Medicaid Costs, The Worst Crunch is Still to Come," *National Journal* 13 (January 10, 1981):44–49.

17. Linda E. Demkovich, "States May Be Gaining in the Battle to Curb Medicaid Spending Growth," *National Journal* 14 (September 18, 1982):1584–1588.

18. Ibid., 1586.

19. Suzanne Powells, "Consequences of Medi-Cal Contracting Unknown," *Hospitals*, 57, No. 7 (April 1, 1983): 23.

20. Walter J. Unger, "HFM Interview: William A. Guy: California Charts a New Competitive Course," *Healthcare Financial Management* 12 (December 1892):60–74.

21. Davis and Millman, *Health Care for the Urban Poor.*

22. Ibid.

23. The New York Times, May 8, 1983.

24. The impact of the shift to block grants was pronounced in St. Louis. The reduction and restructuring of federal assistance resulted in an initial 47 percent reduction in maternal and child health funds (later partially restored so as to produce only a 25 percent loss) and a 93 percent reduction in federal moneys available for the city's lead poisoning prevention program.

25.   Voluntary agencies indicated in a survey taken by the United Way of Metropolitan St. Louis that "since 40 percent of agency dollars had previously come from federal grants, most expected their revenue to decline and were already discontinuing programs" [figures from: John Herbers, "St. Louis Struggles With Federal Cuts," *New York Times*, October 20, 1981: A8 (cited in Davis and Millman, 184)].

26.   Conservation of Human Resources, *The Expanding Physician Supply, Report I: Agenda For a Physician Supply Monitoring Project* (New York: Columbia University, March 1980), 74.

27.   American Medical Association, *Physician Distribution and Medical Licensure in the U.S., 1976* (Chicago: AMA, 1977); and American Medical Association, Center for Health Services Research and Development, unpublished data for 1981.

28.   Shapiro, et al., *Relationships of Resources* (cited in Davis and Millman, 184).

29.   Figures taken from American Hospital Association, *American Hospital Association Guide to the Health Care Field,* 1979 and 1981 Editions, (Chicago: AHA, 1979 and 1981).

5

The Process of Change

This chapter will discuss the change process involved in accomplishing the modifications in the local public health service delivery system proposed by the Municipal Health Services Program (MHSP) in each of the five participating cities. An effort will be made to identify factors in the local environment which facilitated or hindered local health leaders in attempting to reform the existing system.

The program models originally described by the cities in their grant applications underwent significant alterations during the course of implementation. These modifications were responses to the realities of funding, bureaucratic structures, interest-group pressures, and utilization patterns. Some modifications took place during negotiations with the Robert Wood Johnson Foundation over program details prior to actual implementation. Others were devised early in the program as obstacles or opportunities were encountered in the original work plan. Yet other changes occurred much later as either the funding or political environment changed or as incipient conflicts which had been muted in the early stages erupted into irreconcilable differences.

Elements of Local Government and Health System Structure

At the local level, there are a number of generic characteristics of the health care environment which have notably influenced the implementation of the MHSP. Perhaps the most important characteristic is the local government structure and the locus of responsibility for health services in each of the five cities. One argument for decentralization of responsibility for policy and service provision from the federal government is that the variability in structure and philosophy at the local level inherently implies a laboratory for testing different approaches to problem solving and the opportunity for natural experiments in service delivery and financing. The settings for the demonstration projects of the MHSP certainly fit this experimental construct.

Public Sector Health Structure

Among the five study sites, it is possible to identify four different types of structure and responsibility for health services defined by jurisdictional authority. In two cities, Baltimore and St. Louis, the municipality has legal responsibility for both public health and public hospital services. This model is common to older cities and to the industrial northeastern and midwestern cities. It is notable that neither of these cities is a subunit of any county jurisdiction, holding instead independent status. The other three study cities—Cincinnati, Milwaukee, and San Jose—are contained within overlying countries, usually sharing some responsibility for financing or delivering health services. These three cities, however, exemplify three different models. In Cincinnati, the city is responsible for public health services, but the public hospital, which earlier was a function of the municipality, is now the responsibility of state government and serves also as the principal teaching facility for the University of Cincinnati College of Medicine, a state institution. Overlying Hamilton County operates a separate public health department to serve county residents outside Cincinnati's boundaries. The city of Milwaukee operates a municipal public health department, but the public hospital is the responsibility of Milwaukee County, a third model. The county hospital is located outside the Milwaukee city limits, leading to access problems for inner-city patients. The fourth model is found in San Jose, where the city is responsible for neither public health nor public hospital services. California law vests these responsibilities in county government; therefore, Santa Clara County rather than the city of San Jose operates both the public health department and the public hospital.

Given a strategy of improving municipal health services for inner-city residents by linking public health and public hospital activities, it would appear that chances for success might be greater when both agencies are the responsibility of the same jurisdiction. Ultimately, the health department/public hospital linkage was never fully realized in any of the five cities. Bureaucratic obstacles were responsible for some modifications in the proposed program models, or at least for the failure to pursue aggressively certain intrinsic goals. The two major areas in which essential model modification due to bureaucratic obstacles can be said to have occurred are those of the proposed close integration of clinic primary care with public hospital specialty and inpatient services and the related objective of securing public hospital admitting privileges for clinic physicians. Even in St. Louis, where the health division and hospitals division are combined within

a nominally unified department, historic distrust between the two bureaucracies prevented any full-scale integration of services. Referral arrangements were weak, varying by medical specialty and depending upon the
personal relationships of individual clinic physicians with hospital physicians, some of which were strengthened and formalized as the MHSP progressed. Nevertheless, the projected admitting privileges never materialized.
The public hospital remained a relatively uninterested academic enclave in
Cincinnati, although the new health commissioner was able to negotiate
limited admitting privileges for clinic staff. In Milwaukee and San Jose, not
only separate bureaucracies but separate jurisdictions complicated the
issues of hospital/clinic cooperation. The hospitals simply had no motivation to participate: there were neither financial nor programmatic incentives for them to undertake the prescribed roles. In Baltimore, the initial
active role in the MHSP of the private physician group, which exclusively
staffed the public hospital, promised a close relationship. However, disputes
among the physician group, the health department, and the hospital
administration led to the separation of the physician group from the MHSP
and thus a modification of the relationship with the public hospital. The
physicians with whom the program subsequently contracted for services
were affiliated with a variety of voluntary hospitals as well as with the public hospital. Bureaucratic conflicts were also an issue in Milwaukee, where
the staffs of the city health department and county academic medical center
could not see eye to eye on program implementation. Early in the program
the health department, which was the grantee, attempted to force the
county to meet its demands by simultaneously negotiating to replace them
with other provider groups and, in fact, eventually recruited a private physician group to participate in the program.

Moreover, inter-jurisdictional conflicts were major hindrances to health
department/hospital cooperation in both Milwaukee and San Jose. The
need to involve more than one jurisdiction added several degrees of complexity to the program, primarily because multiple bureaucracies and political structures had to be motivated to approve program organization and
expenditures. Each new participant required the demonstration project staff
(generally located in the city health department) to invest an exponentially
increased amount of time and effort to move the project along. In
Milwaukee, the county supervisors were grappling with large operating
deficits in the public hospital budget at the same time that they were being
asked to sponsor primary care services which would also result in a net
deficit from their point of view. The Milwaukee municipal health
department directly funded only the preventive services component at the
MHSP sites. An array of other providers were to share the physical facility
but to deliver and manage their services individually. The county hospital
had no real incentive to continue its participation. Inpatient referrals did
not materialize and county physician, nursing, and administrative staff were
hostile to city public health nursing and administrative personnel. The billing and financial reporting tasks required under the Medicare waiver
presented problems for the county financial managers because the compu-

terized billing system in place had no provision for the formats required, and all transactions had to be done manually—a costly procedure. The county felt that accounting costs outweighed benefits of the waiver. Eventually the county's budgetary pressures led to the supervisors' decision to close the largest, best-established clinic site despite the city's offer to fund several financial and clinical staff positions. While it is clear that budgetary and professional-domain issues influenced the outcome, the multiplicity of jurisdictions involved was responsible for the long delays in implementation progress and for much of the difficulty in resolving conflicts and correcting problems.

Jurisdictional problems also existed in a somewhat modified form in San Jose. The county public health department was at no time intimately involved in program implementation, despite the integration late in the project of a health department clinic with the demonstration. Jurisdictional conflict arose because the city was the grantee and the moving force behind the program while the county provided all public health services and had financial and legal responsibility for hospital care. As in Milwaukee, the San Jose county hospital was operating with a deficit and had little to gain from participation in the MHSP, since ambulatory care services also generated a net deficit. The county declined any financial responsibility for the MHSP although the director of its public hospital did serve as project director. In order to move the project forward in its early days, the city was forced to establish a steering committee, with membership from all the interested and responsible agencies, to agree upon recommendations to those groups with legal authority to act: the city council, the county board of supervisors, and the county executive. The jurisdictional issue was further complicated because actual providers of clinic services were independent community health centers with governing boards of their own. All these groups, as well as separate community advisory groups established for the new clinic sites which were independent of the parent clinics' governing boards and management, were represented on the steering committee. The mayor's office was the source of strongest program support, but this support was philosophical rather than operational. The city and the county argued at length as to where the financial responsibility for deficits or postdemonstration funding lay, and neither was willing to assume the burden. Disputes over proper management of the program and provision of services by the community subcontractors dragged on for protracted periods because of the lack of a single recognized point of authority and responsibility. The large number of participating interests led to highly politicized conflict and fragmentation which were not amenable to easy resolution. Thus in both Milwaukee and San Jose, progress toward actual delivery of services was impeded by the diversion of staff time and effort to addressing the conflicting interests of multiple participants or simply energizing and synchronizing several bureaucracies at one.

It should not be assumed that St. Louis and Baltimore had no problems by virtue of the municipality's authority over both health and hospital departments. Even nominal unification of these agencies under one department, as in St. Louis, did not guarantee mutual activity or cooperation. In these two cities, the obstacles to cooperation were professional domain conflict and budget deficit stress. The course of the MHSP demonstration witnessed the launching of initiatives by the mayors of both Baltimore and St. Louis to discontinue municipal operation of the public hospital. While neither of these cities was able to transfer responsibility upward to a county or state jurisdiction, Baltimore set up an independent nonprofit organization which opted for management by a private teaching hospital. The degree of continued city subsidy was not clearly specified by the close of the demonstration period. St. Louis, projecting a $30 million deficit for FY 1984, examined several alternatives for its one remaining acute care hospital after the mayor threatened to close it by late 1983. Initial hostile reactions from political and community leaders and the media prompted the mayor to establish another health care study committee. Options for service to the indigent that were considered by the committee and independently by the mayor included contracting for inpatient care with private hospitals, building one new public hospital to serve both city and county residents, and building a new hospital to be managed by a private, nonprofit corporation. All of the alternatives advanced to date carry major financial or political obstacles. Therefore, initially the city concentrated its efforts on regaining accreditation for the existing public hospital for the immediate future while a reconstituted mayor's committee with more political leaders explored further hospital options which might gain community approval.

Qualified accreditation for the hospital was regained on December 16, 1983, but on the same day, the St. Louis University Medical School gave two-year notice of its intent to end its affiliation with it. The medical school stated that staff shortages and the city's lack of commitment to the hospital made it impossible to conduct clinical programs at City Hospital. With St. Louis University Medical School preparing to withdraw, the mayor persuaded the city's budget authority and the board of aldermen to contract with National Medical Enterprises, Inc. of California to manage the municipal hospital. Interestingly, this contract and the factors which motivated it produced an institutional change which MHSP had been unable to accomplish: administration of the MHSP centers was transferred from the health division to the hospital division. Whether this will effect real integration of the health centers and the hospital system in not yet clear. Chances for such integration may be influenced by the fact that the former head of the MHSP demonstration is now acting director of the department of health and hospitals.

Only in Cincinnati did the public hospital, despite its control and operation by a separate jurisdiction, come close to establishing the desired linkages with the health department's clinics. The hospital had been transferred from municipal to state auspices under the parent medical school's control before the city was faced with unsupportable operating deficits. Cincinnati also was the one demonstration city where the municipal health department had a strong established record as a provider of primary care in neighborhood clinics prior to the MHSP. The degree of change required by the MHSP was slight, the city had no hospital crises to distract attention from primary care, and the health department had both strong leadership and a supportive city council.

The Role of the Mayor

Strong political, professional, and managerial leadership was critical to MHSP implementation in each city—at least at intervals—to resolve conflicts or expedite action. In some cities, leaders of neighborhood groups played significant roles as advocates or critics, but community involvement, with the exception of San Jose, was not as extensive or relevant as the original design had anticipated.

Political leadership, it was expected, would be centered in the mayor, whose support would move the health and hospitals bureaucracies to rapid action, garner community involvement, and convey to the professional community a sense of status and respectability for the program. In addition to personal style, predilection, and competing commitments, the influence that mayors actually brought to bear on the program was contingent upon structural factors, and the outcomes were not easily predictable. Structurally, the mayor's influence is related to the degree to which public health and hospital services are controlled by city government, and to the formal powers vested in the mayor's office.

Baltimore and St. Louis represent cases in which both the health division and the public hospital are direct mayoral agencies, so the strongest mayoral influence may be expected here. In Cincinnati and Milwaukee, the health department is a city agency, but the public hospital is operated by state government and county government, respectively, and is, in Milwaukee, the primary teaching facility for a private medical school. Thus, in these cities the mayors have no direct influence over hospital participation and can be expected, at best, to exercise personal political persuasion over the hospital's actions. San Jose's city government has responsibility for neither public health nor public hospital services, both of which are the province of county government. The mayor of San Jose exercises no control over the health services structure, and is limited to a role of advocacy with other officials.

The second measure, formal power of the mayor's office, provides a similar range in degree of potential influence. The mayoralty in Baltimore is a formally strong office, with extensive appointive power, control over the board of estimates which formulates the budget, and greater strength than the city council. In addition, the incumbent is popular and highly visible and prefers a style of active personal involvement in city projects. Baltimore has by far the strongest mayoralty of the five cities. St. Louis, while next in direct mayoral control over health and hospital services, is a city with a weak mayoralty, with few appointive positions, a stronger board of aldermen, and a requirement that budgetary decisions be shared equally among the mayor, the comptroller, and the aldermanic president. Similarly,

Milwaukee has a weak mayoralty with budgetary power shared by the mayor and a variety of special boards and commissions. San Jose and Cincinnati both have formally weak mayoralties, with actual administrative control vested in a city manager. In San Jose, the mayor has greater political visibility than in Cincinnati since the office is filled by public election, whereas the mayor's position is simply a rotating slot among the city council members in Cincinnati.

A final determinant of mayoral influence is the mayor's specific personal commitment to the program of interest, and its place in the hierarchy of other issues which compete for official attention. The mayors of Baltimore and San Jose both identified themselves strongly with the MHSP after initial problems in launching the project led to a request for their intervention as problem solvers. The two mayors to hold office in St. Louis devoted attention to the MHSP primarily as one element in the context of the tortuous budgetary and political challenge of providing health care to the indigent in a fiscally distressed city. At the time the MHSP was initiated, the incumbent mayor was convinced of the need to close one city hospital, Homer G. Phillips, because of the decline in the city's economy and its population, and therefore wholeheartedly embraced the MHSP plan to expand primary health care through municipal clinics as a legitimate redirection of dwindling health care resources. After black voters defeated him for reelection over the Homer G. Phillips issue, his successor initially threatened to terminate MHSP operations as he struggled to balance the municipal budget and reopen Homer G. Phillips Hospital in compliance with his campaign pledge. The new mayor's acceptance of the MHSP increased as his term of office progressed, and it became apparent that it was impossible for the city to reopen Phillips and problematic even to maintain the one remaining public general hospital. In the spring of 1983, the mayor announced his intention to close this remaining hospital by November 1983, a decision he was later forced to rescind for want of a feasible alternative. During the early implementation phase of the MHSP, Cincinnati's mayor was supportive, especially in budgetary decisions, but was not actively engaged in the program. Subsequent mayors demonstrated little direct involvement. Milwaukee's mayor exhibited less personal interest or involvement than any of his colleagues and perceived the MHSP mainly as an extension of a favorite preventive health care project of his.

Whether the mayor involved himself at all in the project seems in each case to have been contingent upon his personal interest. The formal power of his office and the lines of authority within the health care structure determined the nature of that involvement and the degree of success. Baltimore's interested and powerful mayor resolved conflicts and expedited action and can be said to have played a major role. Despite her strong interest, San Jose's mayor was able to move only indirectly and slowly by building a political constituency for her attempts to resolve disputes among multiple actors. Milwaukee's mayor, had he become involved, might have been able to resolve interjurisdictional conflicts. The successive mayors in Cincinnati did not engage themselves in problem solving at any time.

The Role of the Medical School

A second major generic factor in the local environment is the role of a medical school and its teaching programs in the operation of the public hospital and its effect on relationships with the public health department and neighborhood clinics. It appears that a very strong medical school involvement in the public hospital serves as a force to guarantee the survival of the institution, although the facility's governance may shift from direct municipal control. The two public hospitals with extensive medical school ties were Cincinnati General and Milwaukee County, each of which was the primary teaching affiliate of the associated medical school. The sophisticated tertiary care services and educational programs generated public hospital costs that were higher than those of voluntary community hospitals in the area, a source of controversy, especially in Milwaukee. The focus on tertiary services was also criticized by advocates of neighborhood-based primary care, and in fact the teaching centers had difficulty responding to the needs imposed by the establishment of community clinics. The turf conflict between medical school staff and prevention-oriented public health staff was fierce in Milwaukee. Specialty-oriented physicians familiar with OPD clinics did not buy in easily to a health-team approach. However, the integral role of the medical school resulted in the transfer of Cincinnati General Hospital to more secure state governance before the MHSP began, and the prestige and power conferred on Milwaukee County's hospital by its relationship with the Medical College of Wisconsin served to protect it despite severe financial pressures during the course of the demonstration. The county maintained its commitment to the hospital, although it is possible that a shift to Wisconsin state governance may occur in the future.

The public hospitals in Baltimore, St. Louis, and San Jose, while providing many tertiary-level and specialized services common to public facilities serving as teaching hospitals, were not the primary teaching affiliates of the medical schools with which they were associated. Over the course of the MHSP demonstration, Baltimore City Hospitals, and, to a limited extent, St. Louis's public hospitals either lost whatever political constituency they had had previously or succumbed to stronger pressures in the community to reduce municipal subsidies for hospital care.

In Baltimore, the change was proposed without much public interest and with no protest. Although the formal shift in governance was from municipal control to an independent voluntary board, the de facto administrative shift was to management by a group connected with Johns Hopkins Hospital, and the arrangement was openly described as a "transfer" from the city to the private organization, with the city subsidizing uncollected debts up to $12 million over several years. The transfer was intended to be completed by the beginning of FY 1984, leaving Baltimore with no municipal hospital, although the facility would continue to operate as a voluntary community hospital. In essence, the influence of the medical school is reflected in the nature of Baltimore's resolution of its wish to withdraw from municipal hospital operations. The early structure of the MHSP in Baltimore provided for medical staffing of the clinics by physicians from the group that staffed the city hospital. This arrangement effected a close relationship to the hospital and since the physicians were also faculty members of the Johns Hopkins University School of Medicine or the University of Maryland School of Medicine, a degree of medical school influence. The physician groups in Baltimore, although members of teaching faculties, were more oriented toward group practice and community medicine goals than were staff of the public hospitals in the other cities. The public hospital link, however, foundered rather early in the course of Baltimore's MHSP, when irreconcilable differences over contract terms arose between the original physician group and the central administration of the program. The physician groups that succeeded them had ties to several voluntary hospitals and to a family practice residency program at the University of Maryland, which did maintain some medical school influence at one clinic site.

St. Louis operated two public general hospitals at the beginning of the MHSP. The hospitals had severe budgetary problems and successive special studies had recommended closing at least one of the two. The involvement of two medical schools at City Hospital Number One contributed to its choice as the surviving institution. Homer G. Phillips Hospital, traditionally a national training site for black medical residents at a time when there were few other choices, was closed. The mayor's intention to close City Hospital Number One as well prompted several alternative proposals, all of which continued to involve the St. Louis University School of Medicine as the major source of medical staffing. (Washington University Medical School had previously withdrawn from all but the neurology program at City Hospital Number One.) The involvement of the medical school was one of several factors which preserved the status quo in St. Louis' public hospital services for the indigent, despite a multitude of threats.

Unfortunately, neither medical school's relationship was as close to the health division as it was to the hospital division, although both have had extensive ties with freestanding federally funded health centers in St. Louis and with a variety of neighborhood-based health care programs. Most medical school faculty at City Hospital Number One are generally unimpressed with and, at times, openly critical of the quality of medical care delivered in the health division's health centers, a factor that has militated against the establishment of an admissions link between the health centers and the city hospital. On the other hand, health division administrators have insisted upon controlling the assignments of their own physician staff, and have therefore resisted unified medical staffing for the health centers and the city hospital, which would undoubtedly have resulted in the transfer of authority over physicians to the hospital division and possibly to the medical school. Since the medical school is ending its affiliation with City Hospital, and private management is taking control of both neighborhood health centers and the public hospital, many of the issues cited above may be moot. On the other hand, new problems such as recruitment of medical personnel and provision of quality public health care are likely to emerge.

Santa Clara County Valley Medical Center was one of a number of teaching affiliates of Stanford University School of Medicine. The medical school had virtually no involvement in MHSP activities because the hospital staff had only a minimal role. Valley Medical Center's stability as a public general hospital was assured more by virtue of the state mandate that the county serve as guarantor of care for the indigent than by its medical school ties. Another source of stability for Valley Medical Center was its support by community groups. In periods when county officials considered the potential closure of the county hospital, active, vocal support from many community groups was instrumental in keeping the hospital open. The need to maintain community approval led the hospital director to avoid conflict with community clinics in his simultaneous role as MHSP project director, when other local officials and the community advisory groups for the satellite clinics were actively criticising a parent clinic. Valley Medical Center was subject to public criticism for budget deficits early in the course of the MHSP, but the facility was substantially turned around by a new director, between 1979 and 1981. The hospital, however, came under increasing pressure following the enactment of new state health legislation in 1982, which made counties responsible for the care of medically indigent adults and established price competition for Medi-Cal contracts. These pressures were the dominant concerns of the hospital director/project director in the latter period of the MHSP.

The Involvement of the Private Sector

Another important factor at the local level in several of the demonstration cities was the growth of private sector participation in the MHSP. This development is a key facet of the organizational dynamics of the program that was not anticipated in the original Johnson Foundation design. Among the most potent interest groups that shifted program parameters were physician groups and voluntary hospitals.

The MHSP was originally conceived as a partnership between public health and public hospital departments. Among its goals was the stabilization of an underutilized, financially stressed public hospital by providing a predictable flow of inpatient referrals from the neighborhood clinics and by redirecting primary care patients from the crowded and costly emergency room and outpatient department. However, the public sector in at least two of the cities which received awards initially anticipated and encouraged private sector involvement. Funding was predicated upon a modification of the proposal to focus on the public hospital instead.

For example, San Jose's original proposal called for the provision of services at its downtown clinic by a voluntary hospital through its medical group. This arrangement did not materialize. The independent community clinics which subcontracted to provide services for the MHSP, however, did have ongoing relationships with voluntary hospitals which predated the demonstration project. Although the MHSP was not directly involved as a contractor with these hospitals, these relationships implied the use of voluntary hospitals as backup facilities for certain inpatient services for its contractor community clinics. These were established referral relationships which it was not easy or opportune to disrupt, although the administrators of the county hospital would have preferred to see more of the inpatient referrals from the MHSP clinics directed to the public facility as the original concept predicated. Late in the project, a major voluntary hospital proposed to enter the MHSP as the provider for one of the satellite clinics. The community clinics themselves, the direct providers of MHSP services in San Jose, were freestanding nonprofit organizations, independent of the municipality and the county, although each received substantial federal, state, and/or county funds.

Baltimore's proposal described a community medical center model based upon staffing by a private physicians professional corporation. The private nature of the group was tempered by its role as the medical staff of the municipal hospital, but this relationship can be seen as part of a long-term shift of the public hospital to private governance; the formation of the private professional corporation by former municipally employed doctors was an early step in this process. The original MHSP proposal stressed the goal that the health centers become self-supporting and suggested the possibility that they would become private entities independent of the city at the end of the demonstration. The Baltimore MHSP administration has indeed worked to accomplish this goal, which is consistent with a Baltimore tradition of redevelopment projects through public/private cooperation and the creation of nonprofit, trustee-managed agencies to accomplish objectives which would be difficult in the context of civil service regulations and bureaucracies. The Baltimore program also showed the influence of voluntary hospitals interested in protecting or expanding their outpatient (and referral) markets. One MHSP clinic is directly affiliated with a community hospital which exhibits intense interest in securing all referrals for inpatient care. As noted earlier, in Baltimore the two private physician groups have referral relationships with a variety of voluntary hospitals, as well as admitting privileges at Baltimore City Hospitals.

In Milwaukee, overt pressure developed from inner-city voluntary hospitals for a share of both Johnson Foundation funding and the patient market. The strongest interest came from a teaching institution whose services were in direct competition with those of Milwaukee County Hospital. This voluntary hospital had been pursuing satellite ambulatory care programs and had obtained an Urban Health Initiative grant in partnership with a community-based organization. Milwaukee accepted the clinic as a fourth MHSP site in which the city health department placed a separate preventive services component to be "coordinated" with the primary care services.

The existence of previously established referral relationships between community clinic staffs and voluntary hospitals was one factor which encouraged the expansion of MHSP parameters to include the private sector. Equally important, however, was the fact that in most of the cities the

voluntary community hospitals were concerned with their ability to maintain adequate occupancy levels and felt the need to compete for inclusion in
any ambulatory care venture that might capture potential markets for inpatient referrals. Only in St. Louis and Cincinnati did voluntary hospitals not
overtly seek to participate. The national program staff liberalized the rules
to include voluntary hospitals as full-fledged participants in Baltimore,
Milwaukee, and San Jose, at least as backup facilities for individual clinics.
Even in Cincinnati, a voluntary hospital was responsible for all pediatric
referral services due to its relationship with the public institution, which
regionalized its pediatric services at the neighboring private facility. By the
last year of the demonstration, San Jose had determined to end its contract
with one community health center as an MHSP provider and made the
decision, which was later revoked, to transfer the contract to a voluntary
hospital which previously had not been involved in the program. Thus, by
the fifth year the MHSP had been transformed from a public sector experiment to a public/private partnership in three of the five cities.

In all five MHSP cities it appears that voluntary hospital strategies to
improve occupancy rates were successful, at least through 1980. Voluntary
short-term general hospital admissions increased from 1978 to 1980 in the
five cities despite falling population in all but San Jose. Total bed capacity
in such facilities decreased slightly in St. Louis and Cincinnati, increased in
San Jose and Baltimore and remained stable in Milwaukee. (St. Louis
reduced it public short-term beds over 50 percent, Milwaukee about 20 percent, and San Jose under 5 percent, in the same period. Baltimore and Cincinnati remained unchanged.) The general stability of voluntary hospital
admissions may be explained by more aggressive hospital marketing strategies in both the central cities and the suburbs, by an aging population,
and by increases in the physician supply in these locales.

The private sector was also involved through the participation of private
physician groups in some cities. In Baltimore and Milwaukee, the MHSP
has been directly affected by the growth of physician groups. Baltimore originally planned its program around the services of the Chesapeake Physicians Professional Association (CPPA). The CPPA was formed as part of a
strategy to reduce hospital costs, improve the quality of patient care, and
maintain the teaching programs based at the public hospital. The group
continued to have faculty appointments for all its members at Johns Hopkins or the University of Maryland medical school. The CPPA was able to
provide hospital medical services at a lower cost to the city than it had spent
previously. As staff for the public hospital, the group was key to Baltimore's
original program model. Though the public hospital was located in the
MHSP target area, the local populations tended to use voluntary hospitals.
One of the goals of the MHSP was to enhance the public hospital's role as a
community facility for the target population via "private" practice by the
physician group. Conflicts over control of the program which arose from
the start among the health department, the CPPA, and the public hospital
administration led to the withdrawal of the original contractor. The CPPA
group was replaced by two new groups, each of which draws heavily on

young physicians just completing residencies in Baltimore's teaching hospitals. One group, affiliated with the University of Maryland, is a family practice model tied to the university's residency training program. The second is a multispecialty group, many of whom were trained at Johns Hopkins. The Baltimore environment has produced many physician groups, health maintenance organizations, and health center networks, and the MHSP arrangements are partially a product of this local history.

Milwaukee's MHSP also replaced its original provider, the county hospital/medical school contract for physician and support staffing, with a private physician group. This change of providers was more far-reaching, since a role for a private physician group was not included in the original proposal (although health department staff indicate that it had been considered). The public hospital's agreement to provide physician staff was terminated at one of the new Milwaukee sites after three years. It was replaced by a group of young minority physicians, many of whom had recently completed residencies in Milwaukee's teaching hospitals. One group leader had worked in an MHSP clinic while completing his training. The earlier experience of a black physicians' group that had been unsuccessful in its efforts to maintain a neighborhood health center under OEO funding provided useful lessons to the contemporary group, which is organized as a private practice and has contracted to subsidize services to the indigent. When subsidies are exhausted, nonpaying patients will be referred to the county hospital. The role of private physician groups, while certainly self-initiated in both cities, can also be interpreted as the by-product of conflict between public health department and medical school/public hospital staff. Differences of opinion arose about the level of physician staffing, the costs of contracts, and the highly specialized, intensive approach to care. The MHSP administration in both cities, housed in the health department and generally more oriented toward preventive services and community medicine, became dissatisfied with the hospital/medical school affiliated providers and was amenable to the introduction of alternative providers into the program.

It should also be noted that the physician staff at San Jose's Santa Clara Valley Medical Center were organized as a group practice. However, this structure had no relationship to or impact upon the MHSP. During the course of the demonstration, health policymakers from St. Louis made use of the resources of Baltimore's CPPA to explore the possibilities of creating a physician group at their public hospital, but such a reorganization did not materialize during the demonstration period.

The involvement of voluntary hospitals and physician groups was an unanticipated and major modification of the service models originally conceived for the MHSP. This development appeared to be a product of increasing competition among both hospitals and doctors for a shrinking pool of patients in all the cities except for San Jose with its growing population.

The number of nonfederal physicians engaged in patient care in the counties in which the five MHSP cities are located grew substantially from

1976 to 1981, the latest year for which American Medical Association (AMA) data are available.[1] It is likely, however, that physicians are locating in the suburbs rather than in the central cities of these counties. For example, the Missouri State Health Division reported that the city of St. Louis experienced a rise of only 3 percent in the total number of physicians between 1976 and 1982, while the number of physicians in St. Louis County, which excludes the city, grew by 50 percent. While the state's figures differ from those reported by the AMA, the trend is similar. The increases in the supply of patient care physicians reported by the AMA for Baltimore (9 percent) and St. Louis (10 percent) were the lowest among the five MHSP cities, undoubtedly reflecting the lack of suburban areas within these independent city-counties. Hamilton County, Ohio had a reported increase of 23 percent in its physician supply between 1976 and 1981; Santa Clara County, California, 26 percent; and Milwaukee County, 25 percent. Indications of greater ease in recruiting physician staff and, in Baltimore, Cincinnati, and Milwaukee, a predominance of recent graduates of residency programs in the MHSP clinics, underline the greater availability of young doctors.

The Role of Community Interest Groups

Community groups and neighborhood organizations constitute another set of interests which affected program models, mainly in terms of site location but occasionally extending to the service package and even, in some cases, to selection of the providers of care. Community groups were most influential in San Jose, where organized, articulate constituencies of established clinics advanced their own interests, and equally articulate independent community groups lobbied for services for their neighborhoods, sometimes in head-on conflict. Independent groups developed or coalesced around the new clinic sites, closely monitoring their progress. Dissatisfied with the financial management and the quality of care provided by one contractor for services, an established community clinic, they instituted charges of poor fiscal management and compromised quality and, eventually, the contractor was removed from the program. Community input was less strident in the other four cities.

In Cincinnati, patient constituents influenced the decisions on site selection for two clinics that were relocated. Baltimore's mayor perceived the demand of neighborhood constituents for clinics and committed himself to their construction. Milwaukee evidenced relatively little community group activity, other than the efforts of a preexisting community organization as a limited advocate for one clinic and the assumption by another of an administrative role in the program's one private sector clinic. County threats to terminate services at the clinics evoked only moderate community protest.

St. Louis experienced a great deal of community interest, but the issue was the inevitable perception by the black community of a link between neighborhood health care expansion and the closure of Homer G. Phillips Hospital, the black community's sole public source of care prior to the desegregation decision of the Supreme Court in 1954. Black leaders effectively prevented the expansion of a northside municipal clinic as part of the MHSP demonstration in order to avoid unwanted competition with a freestanding black-operated health center that was supported by federal community health center funds. Black community pressure was also instrumental in assuring that the one new MHSP clinic was constructed in the center of black neighborhood growth, rather than in a section populated mainly by elderly whites. Limited activity by small groups of clinic constituents forced the bureaucracy to perform needed renovations, to halt service cutbacks, and to expand some services. These activities succeeded in preventing program reductions which would otherwise have occurred.

In general, community leadership was neither as integral nor as critical to program implementation as had been expected. Had it materialized, one speculates, community support for and utilization of the clinics might have been much faster to develop. San Jose's volatile community clinic environment did reflect a high degree of community interest in the MHSP clinics. As soon as the program was announced, the supporters and administrators of existing clinics competed vocally and vigorously for inclusion in the funding. After satellite clinics were established, individual community advisory groups were appointed which became independent advocates for their own facilities and critics of the leadership of one parent clinic. The new groups mobilized city and county elected officials to support their positions and ousted the parent clinic from one satellite's management. This was a potent example of community leadership. In St. Louis, the Homer G. Phillips Hospital closure issue evoked a high level of community activity. To a degree, black community leaders were energized into advocacy for the neighborhood clinics, but the hospital issue remained their dominant concern. Meanwhile, as a result of the MHSP program, leaders representing elderly white citizens strongly supported the addition of adult medical services to a traditional categorical clinic in their southside neighborhood.

Idiosyncratic Local Forces

In addition to these generic issues, there were also a variety of idiosyncratic factors unique to individual cities which either directly influenced the MHSP or distorted the local health policy environment sufficiently to have an indirect effect on implementation of the demonstration. These idiosyncratic factors have been aptly described by the field associates.

The most telling characteristic of the local environment in Baltimore is:

the central role of politics and personalities. Baltimore has had an exceptionally dedicated and determined mayor in William Donald Schaefer. Recently elected for his fourth four-year term, Schaefer has set the political and administrative tone for the city since 1971. His single-minded dedication to the city's welfare is widely recognized, as is his lack of interest in personal financial gain.

However, the mayor is correspondingly dedicated to controlling most of the major, and many of the minor, policy decisions in the city government. He is very attuned to ways to gain publicity and/or funds for the city, a commitment that can sometimes hinder orderly program development.

The political tradition in Baltimore's bureaucracies prescribes disguising any agency's problems, enduring less than satisfactory employees, trying to secure direct links to the mayor, and 'making do' without complaining publicly. To do otherwise is to be seen as personally disloyal to the mayor, and to risk being frozen out of his favor and political rewards.

The Municipal Health Services Program initially served several of the Mayor's pet interests: glory for Baltimore (as one of a select group of cities), outside money for the city budget, greater leverage over Baltimore City Hospitals, and new programs with which to reward demanding neighborhoods. The MHSP's requirement of a commitment to strengthen City Hospitals and to provide direct health care services was not seen as a significant deviation from the mayor's plans, because it would have only short-term effects. Thus, the program had a mixed agenda from the start, a fact which its history reflects.[2]

No other mayor occupied such an influential role with respect to the MHSP.

The idiosyncratic feature of the Cincinnati MHSP environment is the unique service dimension of the Cincinnati Department of Health.

The department has initiated a service role in the provision of primary care that is atypical of most city and county health departments. As the central actor in the funding and management of all community health centers in Cincinnati, the control point through which federal and state funds for primary and preventive care flow, the health department is the hub of a network of community-based health services, the Cincinnati Primary Care Network. It is one of the few health departments to have historically offered a comprehensive range of services to its constituents, operating fourteen health centers, either directly or by contract, prior to the inception of the MHSP.[3]

Given that Cincinnati had already developed a network of primary care clinics that conformed to the model described by the Johnson Foundation for the demonstration, the focus of its proposal was on improving the linkages among the clinics and their backup hospitals by means of a computerized medical information system and secondarily, on expanding hours and services at three specified clinics. The computerized information system had been initiated at two clinics under a federal grant received from the Department of Health, Education and Welfare (HEW) in 1975. The Johnson grant was to support the inclusion of additional sites and the development of information subsystems. The computer system was the most important element in the proposed relationship between the clinics and the public hospital.

Slow progress with the computer system and budget overruns in 1978 and 1979 led to great controversy and to the investigation of the health department's management of the computer system by the city auditor and the city detective at the request of the city council and city manager. A December 1979 report of mismanagement and inadequate control of outside consultants led in 1980 to an HEW audit of expenditures. While the audit absolved the health department staff of any wrongdoing, stronger in-house management was required; the department's new commissioner had already taken steps to tighten control.

The controversy over the long delays and high costs involved in implementing the information system caused stress among the many actors involved and diverted staff time and energy from other urgent activities such as acquiring staff and supplies needed for patient care. As a consequence of the desultory implementation of the system, useful medical information that could effectively link the centers and their backup hospitals did not become available during the course of the MHSP demonstration.

The most important program determinant peculiar to the Milwaukee environment was the structural division of local responsibility for health services. The interaction between the city health department staff and the county hospital/medical school staff determined the outcome of the project's design. The MHSP grant was awarded to the city health department, a traditional agency oriented toward prevention and community health nursing (the latter commanding almost half the department's 1982 budget of nearly $11 million). The MHSP clinics offered a variety of services provided by multiple agencies in one building, with no formal, organizational linkages beyond the proposed city nurse-coordinator role.

Primary care was county turf but the grant was to the city with primary care to be provided through an awkward arrangement with the county. The county needed to be wooed but was not. The budget was an example, in that it placed all the costs of primary care services with the county. Grant funds only paid city health department administrative personnel and division of health nurses. In the spring of 1981 when the first city/county breakdown occurred, the city was happy about Foundation assurances that the grant funds not yet expended could be extended into sixth and seventh years. An equivalent of 17 full-time health department staff had salaries paid by the Johnson grant as administrative staff of either the MHSP or the Family Health Clinic in the MHSP centers. The county, with no staff paid by the grant, was losing money. The distribution of funds was known only to city officials. As the county administrator who oversaw the clinics said:

We don't know things like the budget, for example, how much is the current budget annually and who is getting what part of the budget in relation to the services provided. We really don't know that and we don't know how fair all of it is. [4]

The city health commissioner believed that the project would have worked except that the county put administrators in charge of the project whose priorities were with the county institutions, rather than the clinics. County and medical school officials considered the centers as luxury items which delivered few patients to the county hospital, provided little educational experience for residents, and little research opportunity for faculty, expensive luxuries which looked more expensive every day because of the special drain they put on the county tax levy. Whereas clinics on the hospital's campus were budgeted only 15 percent from the tax levy, the MHSP clinics drew 55 percent from this source. Thus DMHS, the county's own clinic, by far the best used of the MHSP sites, was the first to close. [5]

The relationship described in the initial Milwaukee proposal had been dramatically altered by the end of the demonstration, with the termination of county participation in other than a token role at one health center, and with disrupted relations among city health department, county administrative, and medical school professional staff.

St. Louis presents the most far-reaching idiosyncratic local development—the protracted battle over the future of the city's public hospitals. The fiscal pressures that threatened continued operation of public hospitals in other municipalities were more intense in St. Louis, which was scored as the nation's most distressed city in studies of urban hardship in the mid-1970s.[6] A historic legacy of racial segregation (which only Baltimore shared among the MHSP sites) figured prominently in the strong and widespread struggle of the black community for the preservation of Homer G. Phillips Hospital, long a symbol of achievement for that community.

As early as the 1960s, proposals to reduce the city's hospital commitments were advanced, with plans for consolidation, the construction of a single new facility, or ending operations completely. From 1973 on, studies by a series of consultants and commissions recommended closure of Homer G. Phillips, and three successive mayors, Cervantes, Poelker, and Conway, initiated efforts to do so. The hospital was finally closed by Mayor Conway in late 1979 after three years of bitter conflict among the board of aldermen, the mayor's office, the city comptroller, and the black community. However, the mayor was dramatically unseated in the March 1981 mayoral primary by an opponent who promised to reopen Homer Phillips and close City Hospital Number One, the remaining public facility. The new mayor was unable to follow through on his campaign promise, and by early 1983, fiscal reality prompted him to announce unilaterally his intention to close the remaining public hospital in 1983. As previously detailed, the mayor could not implement this either. City Hospital Number One continues to serve the health needs of the city's indigent, though now under private management which must seek professional personnel to replace the departing St. Louis University Medical School faculty and medical students.

The dire financial condition of St. Louis, a result of population loss and deterioration of the economy coupled with an aging infrastructure and a large dependent population, is the underlying reason for the public hospital crises. The political division between the city's leadership and its black citizens who constitute nearly half its population has been intensified by policy choices to eliminate services which cost the city large amounts of tax dollars but are identified closely with the blacks. The public policy agenda has been dominated by the hospital issue for ten years, leaving little room for attention to such less-visible programs as the MHSP.

Unique to San Jose was the role of independent community groups as health service providers and the degree of politicization of decisions related to service delivery by these groups. The San Jose MHSP model involved the provision of health center services at four clinic sites by two preexisting community health centers under subcontract from Santa Clara County. The two established community health centers had been in operation for several years prior to the start of the MHSP. One was a large, multimillion dollar, federally funded center which also had several state health project grants. It had begun to establish satellite clinics, and two of its sites became MHSP participants. The interaction of the administrator and board of directors of this parent organization with the MHSP-required community advisory groups established for the two satellite clinics and with city and county officials resulted in a high level of strife and controversy throughout the life of the project.

The community advisory groups at the two satellite clinics reflected the commonly accepted characteristics of community-based health center boards in California. Their members are openly elected periodically; they meet with their larger constituency; their meetings are open and minutes are circulated; they rely upon their own information; they do not hesitate to ask pertinent questions. In short, they have a power base apart from the director of either clinic. In contrast, judged from this perspective, the parent clinic's board was not a functional community board: it was hand-picked by its director. It was not elected at large, nor did it report to a larger constituency (either a consumer or a community constituency). It did not perform the oversight function that a community board should: it did not ask hard questions of the director and his staff; it relied upon information supplied solely by the organization; it did not seek outside opinion; it did not meet with a large constituency; and it had no way of eliciting opinion from the larger clientele. Its meetings were closed, visitors were not allowed, and minutes of its proceedings were never circulated.
    The relation between the parent clinic and the satellite community advisory groups broke down over substantive issues of services, personnel and finance. The advisory groups, in touch with their constituency, heard of problems encountered in the receipt of services, and translated those concerns into administrative and policy questions. They failed to get satisfactory data or answers to their questions from the staff and board of the parent clinic. They felt that they had the responsibility to ensure the quality of the services, and began the process of publicly raising concerns that ultimately led to the involvement of both city and county elected officials, the courts, and auditors from the state and federal level.[7]

    The advisory groups opened the program to direct public accountability. Their impetus, along with the necessity for the mayor's office to maintain accountability for MHSP grant funds, led to the establishment of the MHSP Steering Committee, a political body incorporating representatives of city and county government and the community groups. This group may be able to play an important role in helping to expedite in Santa Clara County the many new health policy decisions which will have to be made at the local level in California in the near future.

A Slow Start

Following the awards, implementation of the Municipal Health Services Program by the five grantee cities got off to a slow start. It began with a formal planning period in four of the cities, lasting from six months to one year. In the fifth city, the decision to plunge directly into operations resulted in a variety of problems ranging from excessive physician staffing to the lack of any system for billing, collections, and financial management. In the two cities in which the county operated the public hospital, the planning period was used to negotiate agreements and contracts among the various participants in the program. Program structure in these two cities was much more complicated than in the remaining three, involving provision of services by a consortium of community-based clinics, voluntary hospitals, county government, health professions school, and independent organizations. In two cities with strong traditional public health agencies whose commissioners had responsibility for program implementation, the planning period was used to establish procedures for billing and financial management and for medical information, and to recruit clinic level managerial staff. The cities dedicated efforts ranging up to 20 percent of the five-year grant period to formal, funded planning for program implementation; in most cities planning preempted 10 percent of the scheduled five years. This investment appeared to pay off, since financial management in most cities could at least generate bills for services, although collection systems were not sophisticated, and it was difficult to reconcile financial records with other sources of utilization information.

The initially desultory progress in program implementation must be considered in light of two common failings of public sector administration. The first relates to personnel regulations and procedures of municipal or county government, which characteristically can neither hire nor fire employees with alacrity, and which is often not competitive with the private sector in recruitment. The second is the notorious length of time required to accomplish public construction projects, due to both political and procedural constraints. Each of these sets of obstacles contributed to the delays which all five cities experienced in renovating or building clinic sites and in staffing them.

Staffing Constraints

The grant proposal submitted to the Johnson Foundation originated at a different level in each of the five cities, and the source of the proposal influenced the subsequent recruitment or appointment of the day-to-day manager of the program—usually an associate or assistant project director. In three cases, the health commissioner or the director of health and hospitals was designated as project director and hired a full-time subordinate to implement the program. In Cincinnati and Milwaukee, where the proposal had been prepared under the health commissioner's direction, hiring of a full-time manager assumed a higher priority and greater control by the commissioner. In San Jose, where the proposal was initiated by a mayor whose jurisdiction covered neither the health department nor the public hospital, the selection of the program manager, who was employed by the county hospital, was beset by political and bureaucratic obstacles. In Baltimore, a consortium of health department, city hospital, private physician group, and mayor's office representatives developed the proposal, and each group wished to control it; although administration was housed in the health department, these conflicts engendered delays in recruitment and early instability in the position of project director.

The projects were delayed to some degree in each city by the time required for posting available positions and filling them through the civil service system. These delays affected the hiring of lower-level managers, nurses, technicians, and other support staff. Seniority rules, salary limitations (especially in St. Louis), and hiring freezes due to budget cuts (in St. Louis, Baltimore, and Cincinnati) were serious impediments to the prompt acquisition of a competent staff. Bureaucratic infighting in Baltimore caused extended delays by health department administration in approving program positions for hiring. In San Jose, delays in hiring by community-based clinics were due mainly to uncertainty about funding levels from the multiple grant sources on which they depended and to the need to negotiate with community governing or advisory boards over the approval of candidates. When the county subsequently entered the program with its own clinic, budgeting concerns and bureaucratic hurdles resulted in a long delay in hiring new staff.

The recruitment and hiring of physician staff was subject to a somewhat different set of obstacles. In Cincinnati and St. Louis, physicians were employed by the traditional health division, which did not have the earnings or status appeal of either private practice or employment by a teaching hospital. In St. Louis, at the outset of the program, physicians were subject to the city's salary limit of $25,000, which made it extremely difficult to attract qualified personnel. In Milwaukee, physicians were employed by the public teaching hospital, which could offer higher salaries, status, and professional contacts. In Baltimore, the private physician group, CPPA, first staffed the program under contract. Neither Baltimore nor Milwaukee had problems recruiting physician staff, but each had considerable staff turnover in the early stages of the program. San Jose's physicians were hired by the individual community clinics, which sought Spanish-speaking staff to better serve their clientele. This constraint, as well as uncertain funding, created some early delays; later, internal conflict among administrators, board members, and professional staff led to considerable physician turnover. Most of the cities had some difficulty early in the program in recruiting physicians, especially full-time personnel in the primary care specialties they were seeking, including family practice and obstetrics/gynecology. However, as time passed and larger numbers of newly trained physicians became available, recruitment problems eased considerably, but difficulties in staff retention took their place. By the third year of the program, the majority of physicians staffing the MHSP were board certified or board eligible in their specialties, except for St. Louis which relied upon a large number of per-performance physicians with generally more limited credentials.

Thus, different factors contributed to delays in staffing across cities, among position types and among employee categories. Procedural obstacles, budgetary constraints, and political conflicts were the major contributors to these delays.

Site Development Delays

In all five cities, implementation of the MHSP required renovation or new construction for at least two sites; overall, only four or five clinics required no capital investment. In an atmosphere of budgetary constraint in three of five cities, funding for capital expenditures presented a problem. San Jose and Milwaukee were in better fiscal condition, but in these cities nonmunicipal providers were responsible for program implementation. Therefore it was necessary to negotiate county government and/or voluntary hospital or community clinic approval as well as municipal and agency support in order to accomplish the necessary renovation or construction. The funding packages for physical improvement were patched together from state, county, and federal sources including the Urban Health Initiative (Baltimore, Milwaukee, and San Jose), Community Development Block Grants, state categorical program dollars and direct state, county, and city subsidies. In addition, in Baltimore private developers were encouraged to build clinic sites with the promise of a long-term lease of space for health services by the city. Construction of these facilities was to be financed through industrial revenue bonds. However, when their tax deductibility was threatened in Congress, the developer refused to proceed with the project, causing further delay.

It may be that greater delay was incurred due to conflicts over site selection than to problems in securing or expending capital funds. The identification of appropriate and acceptable space for clinics presented difficulties in all cities. St. Louis and Baltimore had the greatest problems in acquiring sites although San Jose had parallel conflicts over the choice of providers and the resistance to treating a target population of the mentally ill, drug abusers, alcoholics, and geriatric patients at a site which also served families. St. Louis and Baltimore were both faced with the need to find adequate space in areas where the building stock was deteriorated. Three new sites were required in Baltimore, and two in St. Louis. Both cities had to resort to temporary trailers for service delivery. Community groups surfaced in each city demanding that the clinics serve their neighborhoods. Baltimore's mayor responded by promising to open clinics in several communities. This necessitated expanding the program to five sites from four and shifting the initial locations. In some cases, the city had to obtain title to older buildings and have them demolished before clinic construction could begin.

St. Louis renovated a former funeral home, whose original identity evoked community opposition for a time. Each city's health leadership had to mobilize other bureaucracies such as the departments of planning and community development, real estate acquisition, and legal or general services in order to proceed with site acquisition, demolition, and construction. This was inevitably time-consuming. Cincinnati hired a consulting firm to determine the best new location for an older health department clinic. No site could be found which did not exceed both the city's renovation budget and the Johnson Foundation timetable. The city then selected a second clinic for relocation. Community constituencies played a role in slowing the deliberations. Eventually both clinics were relocated, but neither opened until mid-1982, four years into the program.

All five cities experienced implementation delays due to the long period required to obtain capital funds and expend them, as well as to interest group conflict over site location. Disputes among various city agencies, including the comptroller, the budget office, etc., as well as between mayors and city councilmen, and among neighborhood groups, made the decisions about clinic location very delicate or contentious issues. In Baltimore and San Jose, mayors actively intervened in site location decisions. Health department managers often were left to deal with the political problems in the other cities, and temporizing was frequently the chosen strategy for dealing with the conflict.

Although the initial designation of target neighborhoods in the MHSP grant proposals was usually made by mayor's office or health department staff, sometimes incorporating technical and political advice from health agencies and community groups, further maneuvering by interest groups over site location occurred after the grants were received. These interest groups varied from city to city. In several cities, the MHSP was attractive to single groups or coalitions of interests which had already developed related proposals for ambulatory care services through such vehicles as the Urban Health Initiative, health maintenance organizations, or a variety of categorical health or social service mechanisms. Indeed, one criterion for receiving the MHSP award was the degree to which the applicant city demonstrated an ability to assemble funding from diverse sources to support the project. Thus, providers who had received UHI funding in San Jose, Milwaukee, and Baltimore wanted to participate in the MHSP. Voluntary hospitals in these three cities were often involved in the UHI program; their interest lay in capturing MHSP inpatient referrals, especially if a site were located in or near their service areas. Private physician groups were active lobbyists in Baltimore from the beginning, anxious to expand their HMO service areas; later, they became engaged in Milwaukee. Nonprofit agencies were eager to participate in Baltimore, Milwaukee, and San Jose, where subcontractors for various special health and social services were let. All these groups were primarily pressing for inclusion in the program at previously designated sites. Their interests and influence are reflected in the modification of the original design of the program, focussed exclusively on the public sector to a diverse set of models which accommodated voluntary hospitals and other private providers in all the cities except St. Louis.

Other groups intervened in the site selection process for new or relocated clinics. In Baltimore, private developers were particularly interested in two potential clinic sites. The most powerful coalition of interests in site location consisted of the mayor responding to small but visible neighborhood groups. This alliance was most influential in Baltimore, where the health department staff was expected to execute the public promises made by the mayor at community meetings. The mayor of San Jose also took a leading role in negotiating with community clinic leaders and neighborhood groups (as well as county and nonprofit agencies) over where to build or renovate new clinics. St. Louis' mayor, too, became actively involved in promoting particular clinic sites. In both St. Louis and Cincinnati, site choices were related to the relocation and improvement of existing public health clinics: thus, these locational decisions impressed the immediate neighborhoods as win-or-lose issues over what they saw as "their" clinics. This resulted in severe tensions and prolonged negotiation in both cities before acceptable new sites were agreed upon. The health department staffs who were intimately involved in these negotiations may be seen as interest groups seeking to minimize conflict by delay. The health department staff played a similar role in Milwaukee, where it tried to balance county hospital and community group positions while pursuing its own interests. Only in Baltimore did the mayor play an early and important role in settling site location disputes. Everywhere else, a slow negotiating process conducted by health department (or other agency) staff was the rule.

Administrative Turnover

A final element which contributed to the slow pace of program implementation was early managerial instability in most cities. A common pattern across cities was that overall responsibility for MHSP policy and implementation rested with a senior health official. In Baltimore (initially), Cincinnati, and Milwaukee this was the health commissioner; in St. Louis it was the director of the department of health and hospitals; and in San Jose it was the director of the county hospital. Only in Milwaukee did the same official remain in charge. In Baltimore, conflicts between the health commissioner and his staff and the physician group providing services created such delays and difficulties that the mayor moved the MHSP to a special niche within his office under the policy direction of his human services coordinator. Cincinnati's health commissioner left the city for another position early in the project, but was replaced by a former community clinic medical director who was supportive of the MHSP's goals. St. Louis changed mayors and lost its director of health and hospitals halfway through the project and also had a succession of health commissioners. The director of the county hospital in San Jose was replaced fairly early by a successor who was oriented more to internal hospital management than to community clinic operations. This instability of the policy-making leadership made it difficult for program managers to maintain momentum and bureaucratic support during the first years of the program when decisions had to be made on such basic matters as location, providers, and staffing.

Instability of the leadership was further complicated by at least as much turnover among the day-to-day program managers, who generally held the title of assistant project director. Only in Cincinnati did the person holding this position remain in the post throughout the program. Baltimore and San Jose had difficulty filling the position to begin with, and both lost the first incumbent during the first year, as did St. Louis. Milwaukee changed assistant project directors twice later in the course of the program at periods of considerable disruption in the project. The program administrator in each city was the person who actually accomplished day-to-day progress in program implementation. When this position was functionally weak, lost support from the policy leader, or was vacant, implementation stood still. Much of the early delay in implementation can be attributed to the difficulty cities had in employing a strong program manager who stayed in the position long enough to see program goals realized.

It should also be noted that there was considerable turnover in individual clinic administration staff. In San Jose, clinic directors changed repeatedly. In Baltimore, managers were shifted from clinic to clinic. Cincinnati changed directors at the two clinics which were initial MHSP sites. St. Louis and Milwaukee also experienced turnover. This instability affected the rate at which clinics built up utilization and improved financial management. In sum, the MHSP had to overcome persistent managerial turnover in order to reach a fully operational status, and was slowed in its achievement by this instability.

The Role of Leadership

The Municipal Health Services Program required a substantial change in the usual operations of the local public health delivery system and/or the initiation of entirely new delivery mechanisms in each of the five participating cities. It is a truism that a sine qua non for the implementation of basic change or innovation is strong leadership, that is, the interest, support, and an assigned high order of priority of an individual(s) with the political and administrative authority necessary to persuade policy makers to make decisions favorable to the program and to induce bureaucrats to perform promptly the tasks essential for its operation, such as hiring, purchasing, and the like.

Political leadership on behalf of the MHSP was generally exercised either by the mayor or the health commissioner. Mayors in Baltimore and San Jose took an active role in problem solving when disputes among MHSP providers threatened to disrupt the operation of the project in their cities. Milwaukee's health commissioner intervened in similar conflicts among participants. The role of mediator or problem solver in St. Louis was assumed by the director of health and hospitals. Cincinnati's health commissioner served as the negotiator with the public oversight bodies who were critical of the health department for its problems in implementing a computerized medical information system.

Mayors and top health officials tended to become involved only when problems had reached crisis levels which lower-level managers were unable to resolve. These problems generally had serious political implications: in the community (Cincinnati, St. Louis, San Jose, Milwaukee), among powerful participants in the program (Baltimore, Milwaukee, San Jose), or within the health department bureaucracy (Baltimore, Cincinnati, Milwaukee). Understandably, the attention of these top officials was focussed on the

MHSP only at intervals when their clout was clearly needed. Such support was exercised sporadically, with the result that problem solving for the demonstration projects followed an erratic course.

This uneven progress was intensified by the considerable turnover among both policy leaders and day-to-day managers. The projects survived a change of mayor in three cities (Cincinnati, St. Louis, and San Jose), of health commissioner or project director in four cities (all except Milwaukee), of day-to-day project manager in all cities except Cincinnati, and extensive turnover of individual clinic administrators everywhere, especially Baltimore, St. Louis, and San Jose. (In 1984, St. Louis abolished the position of individual health center administrator, replacing the three incumbents with a "travelling administrator" working out of the office of the director of ambulatory care.) Instability of personnel was probably the single greatest impediment to the development of the program.

The individual who served as day-to-day project manager in each city, in most cases the assistant project director, played the key role in program implementation. In Cincinnati this individual was selected from within the health department ranks, in keeping with the grounding of the MHSP in preexisting public health clinics and in the established bureaucracy. Cincinnati's manager was a committed young public health administrator. The first manager of the St. Louis program, the city ambulatory care administrator, was replaced by an experienced former pharmacist who had worked his way up through the hospital division ranks. In Baltimore, progress was stalled due to an ineffective first administrator, and the lack of impetus and organizational skill. In San Jose, a county hospital employee with no community ethnic or political ties was initially selected as manager and encountered substantial opposition. Following these initial failures, a publicized search for a competent administrator from outside the bureaucracy of the health department (Baltimore) or the county hospital (San Jose) was initiated. In each case, a reasonably independent administrator was hired. The new San Jose manager had an appropriate background with community organizations, and the Baltimore recruit was experienced in both hospital and freestanding ambulatory care administration, and became a major force in trying to free the program of its dependence upon the health department in which it was originally based. Milwaukee's health department engaged a former city employee as grant writer and later project manager, an individual with a background in health program planning who was familiar with the various provider organizations in Milwaukee and their leaders. The Milwaukee project, which needed the cooperation of participants from an array of agencies, was originally given semi-independent status within the health department. When the original manager resigned midway during the demonstration, a physician specialist in preventive medicine was recruited from outside to enhance relationships with the county hospital and the medical school, and at the same time the project was brought into the main line of the health department bureaucracy. Internal conflicts subsequently led to the departure of the physician director and to assumption of control of the project by the health department's division of nursing under the direction of a public health nurse of long tenure with the agency.

Project managers based in health department bureaucracies tended to exhibit more conservative administration styles and were less inclined toward dramatic change in operating procedure or program model. Cincinnati's program did not require extensive change, although the development of the computer system and the constraints on resources posed challenges. St. Louis' project managers were forced to operate in an atmosphere of great political and financial stress and uncertainty. The adaptation of their clinics from a traditional public health nursing model to a physician services model meant that they confronted considerable role conflict within the agency as well. The initial management style in Milwaukee was one of political maneuvering, negotiation, and manipulation among the many parties involved in order to unify the various components. Later, after some of the original participants had left the program and the health department nursing interests assumed control, the management style changed to that of a traditional, low-key, public health bureaucracy. San Jose's project manager did not directly oversee the provision of services and functioned relatively independently of any established bureaucracy. She served rather as project grant officer for the individual subcontractors in the San Jose MHSP and as a resource in conflict resolution and community relations. Baltimore's project manager was able to operate more independently than the administrator in any other city. Although the project director was an outsider in Baltimore, his deputy was a veteran of the health department's nursing division. Her experience and connections within the city facilitated hiring and purchasing through a health department bureaucracy that was otherwise hostile to the MHSP because of its independence of the agency's control. Other things being equal, although it may be easier to introduce innovations by circumventing traditional health department bureaucracies (Baltimore), established management structures have the advantage of being resistant to disruption (Cincinnati and St. Louis). However, projects which straddle multiple bureaucracies may face insurmountable obstacles to effective management (Milwaukee and San Jose) despite the best efforts of administrative staff.

Professional leadership was usually vested in the health commissioner or a parallel health services administrator. Particularly in those cities with limited mayoral involvement, the health commissioner was the key political leader as well as the determiner of professional policy (Cincinnati and Milwaukee). The director of health and hospitals played this role in St. Louis, while assisting the mayor in dealing with the hospital closure issue. This position shifted from an incumbent with the traditional M.D. degree to a lay administrator with strong managerial capability when the mayor's office changed hands. A similar transition occurred in San Jose, where the head of the public hospital, a physician, was replaced by a lay executive with no strong commitment to the MHSP. During the last year of the program the county executive was made MHSP project director. A not dissimilar shift was executed by Baltimore's mayor, who moved the project out of the health commissioner's jurisdiction into his own office, under the direction of his politically astute, lay human services advisor. In Baltimore, professional leadership also came from the private physician groups under contract to staff the program, though this input was sometimes contentious and self-serving.

In every city, the relative skill, political astuteness, and energy of the assistant project director were critical determinants of project success. Only in Cincinnati was the original choice for this role capable of effecting progress, probably because he was an established staff administrator familiar with the system and experienced in ambulatory care administration, and the goal of the project was to expand, rather than dramatically change, an existing system. The other four cities suffered from false starts. San Jose saw three incumbents and Baltimore two at the outset, and St. Louis lost its day-to-day leadership during the first year while it was trying to establish a new administrative mechanism. Each program eventually gained momentum, however. Milwaukee had problems balancing the need for clinical and administrative skills, and these difficulties became manifest later in the course of implementation.

In Baltimore, Milwaukee, and St. Louis, the traditional public health clinic staff, as well as the health department bureaucracy, were resistant to the new comprehensive medical service model imposed by the program which placed greater emphasis on physician roles. The outcome of the confrontation varied depending upon the locus of program control. Baltimore's health department, after an early and bitter dispute with the private physician group, lost policy control of the program to the mayor's office but retained jurisdiction over purchasing and the hiring of support staff. The physician group also lost its contract to a competing group, but the medical model prevailed, with support from the independent project director. Milwaukee's health department bureaucracy maintained tight control over the grant throughout and used it mainly to support health department nursing and administrative staff for preventive services at the same time that it negotiated the participation of medical providers who financed the costs of service delivery, including billing and collecting for care, themselves. The public health nursing staff was in frequent conflict with the medical staff that provided primary care, especially at the large downtown clinic, and integration of services was limited. In St. Louis the leadership of the department of health and hospitals firmly espoused the policy of transforming the nursing-oriented public health clinics to a comprehensive medical model, and mid-level managers aggressively pursued this goal. The community health nursing staff lost support both from the central health department administration and at the clinic level; as a result, many community health nurses resigned and their training program was discontinued. The physician-centered primary care model replaced the community health nursing, preventive model of service in the St. Louis municipal health centers. Missouri regulations restricting the scope of nurse practitioners and corresponding limitations on reimbursement for their services encouraged this change.

Budget Pressures

Several of the cities were experiencing severe budget pressures prior to the inception of the MHSP. Financial conditions generally deteriorated in all five in the course of the program's history, with health and especially hospital budgets coming under intense public scrutiny as city and county officials attempted to make ends meet. Although Baltimore could be grouped with Cincinnati and St. Louis as fiscally distressed cities, funding problems generally only caused delays in capital activities and in filling positions but forced no real changes in program model. Since many specialty services were provided in Baltimore clinics by private physicians who, in effect, rented practice space, the city's budget did not alter the provision of care. In Cincinnati and St. Louis, however, budget shortages meant that many ancillary or specialty services (dentures, podiatry, dermatology, eyeglasses, etc.) either were never instituted or were curtailed or discontinued partway into the program. The shortage of funds delayed filling physician places and other slots and caused cutbacks in hours of service in all five cities. In Cincinnati and St. Louis, budget crises resulted in decisions to consolidate clinics, which meant closure of one of the MHSP sites in St. Louis.

Even the two more affluent jurisdictions, Milwaukee and San Jose, were not immune to budgetary problems. Although these involved the county rather than the city budget, the projected health services deficit led to the closing of the largest, best established Milwaukee site and to threats from the county to withdraw completely from the program in 1982. San Jose was forced to close one of its four clinics due to budget deficits experienced by that satellite and its parent, which neither the city nor the county government was willing to subsidize.

Utilization Shortfalls

The final set of program modifications relates to the expansion and contraction of sites or services not planned originally and to the impact that utilization patterns had on these choices. San Jose, Milwaukee, and Baltimore added sites in the course of the program, generally in response to interest-group pressure or as a hedge against falling below the Johnson Foundation's mandated minimum of three sites. Baltimore's fifth site was added both because the mayor strongly supported it and because the program's managers were worried that the fourth site would not be ready by the August 1981 deadline and wanted at least four clinics operational. Milwaukee added a fourth site to accommodate a voluntary hospital/community group clinic with Urban Health Initiative funding that pressed for inclusion. The decision was partly in response to the health department's concern that one or more of the county-staffed sites might fail. San Jose's program managers, in order to cope gracefully with the demands of two established community clinics to establish a satellite in a single target area, divided the area and awarded contracts to both groups for satellites. Later, a fifth site, a county public health clinic, was added as a hedge when one community clinic and its satellite became overextended and underutilized and it appeared that both might close. The satellite did close, bringing the San Jose complement back to four clinics.

Three cities closed clinics, due to a combination of budgetary, utilization, and political factors. In San Jose, a community clinic expended a great deal of capital resources, operating funds, and managerial and professional staff time in establishing a satellite clinic. Utilization did not increase at either the parent or the satellite clinic as quickly as had been projected. To remain viable, the parent clinic had to jettison the satellite, since no other party was willing to subsidize the deficit.

St. Louis was in the midst of both a severe budget crisis and a boiling dispute over closure of a public hospital as it attempted to relocate two public health clinics in new facilities. The budget problems led first to the use of temporary trailers for services, and then to the abrupt elimination of one trailer site at the same time that other, non-MHSP municipal clinics were terminated. The site chosen for completion was the one accessible to the black neighborhoods which had just lost their hospital.

Milwaukee's program was fraught with tension between the city and the county from the start. After repeated threats by the county that it would withdraw, a county budget shortfall provided the stimulus for closure of the largest clinic in the program. Underutilization had constituted a more serious problem at the two newer, smaller sites, but fiscal losses were greatest at the clinic with the highest volume, so politics, utilization, and budget coalesced to force the decision.

Notes

1. American Medical Association, *Physician Distribution and Medical Licensure in the U.S., 1976*, Chicago: 1977; and unpublished data for 1981.

2. Patricia Maloney Alt, "Field Associate Final Report for Columbia University, Conservation of Human Resources: Municipal Health Services Program Evaluation."

3. Albert A. Bocklet, "Field Associate Final Report for Columbia University, Conservation of Human Resources: Municipal Health Services Program Evaluation."

4. Ann Lennarson Greer, "Field Associate Progress Report for Columbia University, Conservation of Human Resources: Municipal Health Services Program Evaluation" (September 1982).

5. Ibid.

6. Richard P. Nathan, et al., *Block Grants for Community Development* (Washington, D.C.: U.S. Department of Housing and Urban Development, January 1977): 158-159.

7. David Hayes-Bautista, "Field Associate Final Report for Columbia University, Conservation of Human Resources: Municipal Health Services Program Evaluation."

6

Lessons and Implications

The preceding chapters have presented a systematic reconstruction of the successive stages of the Municipal Health Services Program (MHSP), from its initial design in the mid-1970s to full-scale operation which was reached in late 1982. A wealth of operating data and detailed process information describing the progress of the demonstration in each of the five participating cities has been reviewed and analyzed thematically; therefore it is not necessary to reiterate, even selectively, the major findings of the evaluation. Instead, this concluding chapter will adopt a different vantage implicit in the question: What are the most important lessons for health care policy affecting the urban poor that can be extracted from the evaluation and what are their implications for future reform efforts?

Before developing these policy formulations we will, however, present our summary assessment of the major successes and shortcomings of the demonstration in terms of the explicit goals that the Foundation and its cosponsors hoped to achieve. These were essentially three in number: to develop under municipal auspices a network of neighborhood-based ambulatory-care centers that would provide a comprehensive program of therapeutic and preventive services and thus improve access to underserved target areas; to effect a shift of both patients and primary care resources from the outpatient and emergency departments of the local public hospital to the neighborhood center in the interest of economy; to establish an organic linkage between the hospital and the neighborhood centers whereby the hospital would provide inpatient and specialized ambulatory services to clinic patients on referral and clinic physicians would receive staff privileges enabling them to attend their hospitalized patients. This was to be accomplished at no incremental cost to local government; in fact, it was anticipated that the unit cost of a neighborhood clinic visit would be less than that to the hospital outpatient department or emergency room and there would be a resultant net savings. The effective reorganization of the extant system achieved in each of the cities will be assessed in terms of feasibility, costs, and quality.

The chapter will then turn to a more general set of issues that confront present and future efforts to improve urban health care:

- Is the attempt to replace the historically divided health department/public hospital system of primary care with a more rationally linked structure of neighborhood-based primary care and hospital-based specialty care politically and economically feasible?
- Can the assumptions of the MHSP continue to serve as valid guides for public health policy, in terms of both program priorities and implementation mechanisms and techniques?
- What are the implications of the social welfare philosophy, fiscal imperatives, and national priorities of the Reagan administration and the Congress for the future of the MHSP and the more general health care objectives it was designed to achieve?
- Conversely, what can be adduced from the experience of the MHSP for the health care approaches that are favored by the conservative Reagan administration?

Finally, we will turn our attention to the more defined area of health care demonstration and evaluation research as seen from the purview of its sponsors: the private philanthropic foundation, which occupies a distinctive role in the arena of social planning and experimentation in the U.S.

Achievements of the MHSP

How closely do the achievements of the MHSP approximate the program goals? If we accept the crux of the demonstration to have been that the development of neighborhood health centers for the provision of ambulatory care to the inner-city poor, in preference to the municipal or county hospital, was both feasible and desirable, there is no way to read the record other than as unequivocally confirming the achievement of this primary objective. The associated objective of the sponsors, to enhance the quality of ambulatory care for patients by providing an integrated program of preventive and therapeutic services at the MHSP clinics, was also accomplished. Clinics which had previously restricted themselves to the traditional public health functions of preventive services or categorical services such as maternal and child care were transformed into comprehensive health centers that were available to the entire local population.

The feasibility of neighborhood-based care is reflected in the clinics' utilization data. From a baseline of 100,000 visits in 1977–78, utilization doubled by 1980–81 and then redoubled in 1982–83 for a total slightly above

450,000. The desultory initial growth was the net result of a number of disparate factors, the most important being the differential growth rates of preexistent and newly established sites and varying utilization trends for ongoing as opposed to added or significantly enlarged services. We can infer from the rapid growth in the latter years of the demonstration a necessary lag in response to an innovative program and the spurt that follows once a critical mass of users is achieved. Another major stimulus to utilization was the introduction of the Medicare waiver at those sites where tradition and/ or geography had previously militated against the elderly.

While the impressive final-year figures are indicators of improved access, without the definitive analyses of the survey by the University of Chicago the sources of the substantial increase in the work load of the demonstration clinics are not precisely known. Preliminary analysis has questioned, however, one of the assumptions of the program: that a substantial segment of inner-city residents were without a regular source of care. Most of the population living in the target areas of the MHSP were found to have access to some alternative health provider, primarily private practitioners, although a minority were dependent on the public hospital or on other public or private sector institutional care.

A second major objective of the program, to effect a fundamental organizational reform in the health care delivery system by reducing and ultimately eliminating the role of the hospital as primary care provider, was more problematic. While the neighborhood centers did enroll patients who had previously been treated in outpatient clinics and emergency rooms of both municipal and voluntary hospitals, there was no evidence of a substantial decline in the utilization of these facilities that was referable to the MHSP. Accordingly, there was no significant redevelopment either of financial or of staff resources from the hospital to the clinics. Although four of the five cities put into place a parallel system of subspecialty and inpatient care for the MHSP clinics, the anticipated staff linkages did not materialize and the familiar duplications and discontinuities resulting from this dualism persisted.

The assessment of access, use, and quality leads directly into the overarching question of costs, efficiency, and the continuing viability of the clinics once the demonstration has run its course. Definitive conclusions are elusive since the Johnson Foundation award funds and HCFA waiver revenues are not yet exhausted and only the future will reveal how many of the clinics will be able to survive when forced to operate without this support. Although the final question of viability must be held in abeyance, selected data are available that bear on these critical economic issues.

In the most recent year, 1982–83, the average clinic cost per visit in four out of the five cities amounted to about $57.70 exclusive of program administration, capital expense, and other costs subsumed within citywide budget categories. In Cincinnati the cost was only a little above $30 per visit, a reflection of the fact that a high percentage of all visits were provided exclusively by nurses.

How does this figure compare with the cost of an ambulatory visit at the municipal hospital? The calculated cost of an ambulatory care visit at the municipal hospital averaged $136, which suggests a savings of 60 percent when patients were seen at a MHSP clinic. But these figures should not be accepted uncritically. As we noted, some items were excluded in calculating the cost of a MHSP clinic visit. Further, the calculated cost of an ambulatory visit to a hospital, any hospital, may be inflated by accounting conventions and the use of the step-down in their computation. Nevertheless, even if it were possible to adjust for these factors, the result would be favorable to the MHSP clinics.

One of the goals of the demonstration was to economize in the use of professional resources by greater reliance on mid-level practitioners in direct service provision to patients. A related objective was through improved scheduling and other efficiencies to reach a productivity level of 4,500 visits per annum for each full-time employee; by 1982–83 the short-fall was modest (4,350), less than 4 percent.

The substitution of mid-level providers for physicians proved more difficult. In three out of five jurisdictions—Ohio, Wisconsin, and Missouri—state practice codes and Medicaid reimbursement regulations placed major hurdles in the way of extensive use of physician extenders. Even more important, however, was the change in the market for physician personnel. At the time that the demonstration was designed, the reimbursement and recruitment of physicians for work in institutional settings in low-income areas, part-time or full-time, was difficult, particularly if the clinic sought to attract graduates of U.S. medical schools. However, as the MHSP progressed, the market eased and with few exceptions the clinics did not encounter major difficulties in hiring the number of physicians that they required. Under these circumstances, there was less motivation to experiment with mid-level providers. Nevertheless, many of the clinics found it desirable, at least selectively, to utilize mid-level providers for particular assignments, particularly well-baby care.

The efficient use of physicians and mid-level providers to deliver the range of services that they offered was only one half of the challenge that the clinics faced. The other was to establish a billing and collection system that assured that they would receive maximum revenues from third parties or from the users themselves so as to reduce the gap between total outlays and total receipts. Both preexisting and new clinics, almost without exception, found difficulty in establishing effective reimbursement and payment systems; however, most have made notable progress in this critical operation.

How did the MHSP fare financially in 1982–83, the final scheduled year of its operation? For the program as a whole, revenues were slightly in excess of $20 million; operating expenses $23.5 million. By far the largest share of the budget (net administrative costs) was met by Medicare, with its contribution of 34 percent, followed by local government, 25 percent, and Medicaid, 12 percent. Other grants, primarily by federal or federal/

state programs such as the Urban Health Initiative and Maternal and Infant Care, amounted to 11 percent; and self-payment, 4 percent. Johnson Foundation support, which was allocated to the operating deficit, contributed 25 percent.

Although there was considerable variability among cities in the relative importance of the several funding sources, depending on the nature of the program and its service population, these summary data underscore the dependence of the clinics on the Medicare waiver which will terminate at the end of 1984; local government allocations; and the Robert Wood Johnson award which terminated in 1983, but has made available unspent sums extending into 1984 and in some cases into 1985.

Even if one assumes that there remains some additional margin for the sites to improve their billing and collections there is little prospect as of now (1983) that they could continue operations at their present level once the Medicare waiver and the Johnson Foundation grant are no longer available to them. We estimate conservatively that perhaps slightly more than half of the presently functioning clinics would be able to survive these combined losses without new sources of support.

Several additional points bearing on the long-term financial viability of the MHSP clinics should be noted. The original design contemplated the possibility that the range and quality of the services that the clinics would provide would attract nonindigent patients capable of paying for their care through insurance and thereby diversify the clinic clientele as well as strengthen its revenue base. This did not occur, surely not to any significant degree. The only qualification to this judgment might be the increase in the Medicare-eligible population but in general the clinics did not include especially large proportions of the elderly.

Perhaps the most tantalizing of the economic questions connected with the MHSP demonstration is to reach an on-balance judgment about what the additional dollars invested by the Johnson Foundation and HCFA (by means of the Medicare waivers) bought in terms of health care benefits for the poor. The findings of the survey by CHAS will speak definitively to this question, but a first approximation seems to be that the existence of the MHSP program enabled many of the inner-city poor to obtain more and better ambulatory health care services. There is initial evidence to suggest that those Medicare beneficiaries who used the centers received less inpatient care than others who used alternative facilities and thereby consumed fewer dollars. The extent to which these savings may have been offset by higher ambulatory care costs is a major question. Beyond the cost factor, it would be desirable to assess whether the broad array of preventive services offered under the Medicare waiver produced a measurable reduction in morbidity among the elderly and if so, whether the effect was substantial or negligible. It is unlikely, however, that this question, which is highly relevant to the current national debate on future Medicare benefits, can be answered.

A simple approach to estimating the value of the benefits resulting from the MHSP demonstration might start with the query: Where would the patients who were treated in the MHSP centers have sought care in the absence of the demonstration and what would have been the total costs of providing them comparable services at these alternative sites? Assuming that the 350,000 additional visits provided by the centers could have been provided elsewhere at a marginal cost of $57 (the average achieved in the final year of the MHSP), incremental costs would have approximated $20 million. If the same output were produced at the average cost of a municipal hospital ambulatory care visit, the total would come to $47 million. The combined five-year contribution from the Foundation and HCFA (via the Medicare waiver) amount to some $38 million.

The foregoing figures are suggestive, not definitive. We conclude that in the absence of the demonstration the total dollar outlays for the care of the inner-city poor would probably have been less; the volume and quality of the services which they received would have been lower; and patient health status and satisfaction *may* have been poorer. While the data do not permit us to quantify, or otherwise estimate, the improvement in health care and health status for the poor that was accomplished, we can infer that the demonstration provided a reasonable return to society for the additional dollars that it consumed.

Lessons

In view of the inherent uncertainties in calculating the economic costs and benefits of the demonstration, it is important to examine whatever clues and guides it offers to the improved formulation of health care policy, particularly in a period when the total flow of public revenues into the system is likely to be seriously constrained. We will now focus on the various lessons that can be extracted from the demonstration for the strengthening of urban health care policy.

To begin at the beginning, the Foundation entered into partnership with the U.S. Conference of Mayors in the belief that the multiple reforms required to restructure the health delivery system and redirect the provision of ambulatory care from the municipal hospital to neighborhood clinics could be accomplished only if the mayor was able and willing to assume a position of leadership in bringing about the complex changes that such a restructuring demanded.

The record is revealing. Only one of the five cities, Baltimore, had a strong mayoralty with control over both the budget and the bureaucracy. In Milwaukee, budgetary and executive powers are widely dispersed in the city government structure; nevertheless, through his skillful personal political strategy, the mayor had achieved control over the budgetary process and the bureaucratic structure. As for the others: the mayor of Cincinnati held an essentially ceremonial office; in St. Louis, the mayor shared power with a comptroller and chairman of the board of aldermen with whom he was forced to negotiate on all contentious issues; in San Jose where responsibility for all health services is a function of the county (in confor-

mity with California statute), the mayor had principally political influence
and no official direct role in the health care system.

In two of the cities—one of them Milwaukee—governed by a politically
powerful mayor the critical health care institution, the public hospital, was
under the jurisdiction of the county. In short, only the city of Baltimore
met the conditions of governance postulated by the demonstration: a
strong mayoralty and municipal control of the financing and delivery of
health care for the poor and indigent. The remaining four cities did not fit
the presupposed model.

The complexities were not limited to formal structure. In the cities with
strong mayoralties, Baltimore and Milwaukee, the incumbent at the inception of the demonstration continued in office in 1983; that was not the case
in St. Louis, San Jose, or Cincinnati.

Nor is strong mayoral commitment sufficient. There is little in the
experience of Baltimore and St. Louis that lends support to the initial
assumption that an interested and concerned mayor would be both willing
and able to undertake the task of reducing resources at the disposal of one
long-standing governmental unit, the city hospital, in order to increase
those of a new health delivery instrumentality, the neighborhood health
center. Even the strongest mayor operates within ineluctable constraints.
First, mayors must stand for reelection, usually every four years. It is a
truism of politics that incumbent politicians who withdraw benefits from a
well-defined constituency, such as hospital employees, will lose more support than they are likely to gain by expanding benefits to neighborhoods,
such as offering improved services. A strong mayor may on occasion challenge his own bureaucracy and risk the ire of neighborhood voters by seeking to reduce or close a municipal hospital but no mayor, no matter how
well entrenched, is likely to expend his limited political capital in this way
unless he is threatened by still less sanguine options.

There is, however, another side to the interaction between politicians and
neighborhood groups which is encouraging for the future viability of many
of the health centers that offer a wide range of services to the urban poor.
Now that the clinics are fully operational and are providing as many as
30,000 to 40,000 visits a year or more, the pressure on local politicians to
find the necessary funds to maintain these sites, at least the stronger ones,
will be very great. The smaller the gap between clinic revenues and expenditures, the more likely that the mayor and his supporters will make a serious effort to find the funds that the larger clinics will need to stay alive.

One of the unexpected developments during the course of the demonstration relates to the interest of various private-sector providers, specifically
voluntary hospitals and private physician groups, in establishing linkages
with the MHSP centers. In Baltimore, where physician care has been consistently provided by contracting with private practice plans, this linkage
was present from the outset. These arrangements have become more
diversified, and at present one private physician group is seeking to become
a capitated provider of services for Medicaid beneficiaries under the state
regulatory authority.

In Milwaukee a group of minority physicians in the inner-city worked out an arrangement with one of the MHSP clinics to provide physician services for their enrollees; the agreement stipulated that a proportion of the clinic patients who had no coverage and could not afford to pay would be treated free of charge.

Turning from physicians to hospitals, in Baltimore, Milwaukee, and San Jose several voluntary institutions located in the inner-city have arranged to serve as backup facilities to one or more of the MHSP centers, partly as a means of bolstering their falling occupancy rates.

These unanticipated developments are noteworthy in light of the growing interest on the part of all levels of government—federal, state, and local—to experiment with one or another form of capitation for the delivery of health care to Medicare and Medicaid beneficiaries. The best prospects for progress along this axis will be through the active involvement of private physician groups in association with selected voluntary hospitals. This does not preclude the possibility that a locality may, under favorable conditions, be able to initiate a capitated system solely through its own efforts and its own resources, but the inherent financial risk and the need for flexibility suggest that serious experimental programs will only be implemented with the active engagement of nonpublic organizations.

The interest of private groups in cooperating with the MHSP clinics may be interpreted as a recognition on their part that in an era of constrained dollar-flows into the health care system, an enlarged flow of physicians into practice, and a likely decline in days of hospital care among insured populations, enrolled Medicare beneficiaries and, under certain conditions, Medicaid patients as well may constitute a valuable addition to their patient pool.

A note of warning must be struck, however. Thus far there has been no unequivocal evidence that a capitation system for low-income groups can succeed financially under conditions that guarantee adequate services of acceptable quality. The two largest experiments at present, those in California and Arizona, have yet to yield trustworthy results. Earlier efforts by prepayment plans to enroll Medicare and Medicaid patients were tightly controlled because of the concern that if the proportion of these patients exceeded 5 or 10 percent of total enrollment, the financial stability of the plan would be jeopardized. Unless government devises a capitation system for the entire population that will include those patients who now use the clinic but have no third-party coverage and no personal resources, a rapid proliferation of capitated plans would have either of two undesirable outcomes: failure of the plans as viable instruments for delivering a satisfactory level of care to all users; or their abandonment of the uncovered poor to seek services elsewhere (most probably at the city hospital) or to suffer deprivation.

Even if the putative savings that result from the reduced frequency of hospital admissions among Medicare beneficiaries who use the MHSP clinics is not offset by a greatly expanded utilization of ambulatory services, it is questionable that potential economics would be sufficient both to compensate for the loss of Foundation support and of revenue from the Medicare waivers and to provide funds for the uncovered enrollees. The nation should have learned by now that, as Dr. Robert Ebert has stated, there is no free health care: when the poor and the indigent receive care at no charge some other group must pay for it. The group least able to bear the burden of such unreimbursed outlays would be the poor and the elderly who have coverage.

There remain a related number of themes that warrant brief discussion if we aim to assess the demonstration as a whole and to distill from it the most important lessons for future policy. The first can be subsumed under the broad rubric of management, marketing, and margins for innovation and adjustment. Over the life of the program, which at peak operated a total of 22 sites in five cities, each with a full-time program director, some 40 or so persons had the opportunity to play a leadership role in the management of an ambulatory care center. They were challenged by the need to become operational as soon as possible and then expeditiously to build up utilization to an acceptable level within what was in most cities a worsening environment for the allocation of additional health dollars. Not all the program or site directors proved effective, but most of them succeeded in the opportunity to implement an innovative program and remained in their positions for a good part, if not all, of the five years. In mastering and resolving the inevitable challenges and crises, they gained knowledge and experience and developed into more competent and broader-gauged health administrators. A reasonable number of these individuals were recruited from minority groups that had restricted opportunities for employment in managerial positions where their abilities could be proved. Thus, one important by-product of the demonstration was the contribution that it made to the identification, assignment, and advancement of a new cadre of health care administrators who demonstrated a capacity to deal with the multiple, often conflicting, forces impinging upon the clinic from the immediate neighborhood and from outside. Any comprehensive balance sheet of the costs and benefits of the demonstration must include an entry on the asset side that reflects this substantial gain in human resources. The full returns of this increment will only be known in the years and decades to come.

Midway into the demonstration, it became apparent that several of the centers were encountering serious difficulties in expanding their utilization sufficiently to bring their potential revenues into balance with their costs. Hence the central administration began to impress upon the programs the critical need for "marketing," that is, more aggressive efforts to inform various inner-city groups of the existence of the newly established and/or expanded clinics and the potential benefits of utilizing their program of health care services. Information was disseminated broadly about specific "marketing techniques" that had been employed successfully by one or more of the sites; lagging sites were encouraged to seek consulting assistance for their particular problems, and training sessions were held to help the sites to hone their marketing capabilities. Despite these efforts, three sites failed to achieve a level of utilization that justified their expenditures and were terminated. Some others, even after receiving technical assistance with marketing, encountered difficulties in meeting designated targets and thus their future was precarious. These were, however, in the minority.

From the vantage of an outside evaluator, rather than that of a program manager, two aspects of this marketing effort should be noted even if their assessment remains equivocal. The first raises the issue whether in the context of the demonstration as a whole, such strong emphasis on marketing to increase the utilization of the participating centers was an unequivocal good. The resultant increase in demand for services could reflect a number of factors: a shift of patients from other providers to the neighborhood center; the enrollment of unserved patients; or the provision of additional services to previously enrolled patients. In the absence of definitive information, a reasonable assumption is that the first and third factors accounted for most of the increased utilization. There is, however, disutility in the proliferation of service agencies that compete for the same population; therefore to the extent MHSP centers siphoned patients from other providers, their growth may or may not have been a social benefit. On the other hand, the fact that enrollees of the centers were encouraged to use more services was probably, though not necessarily, a social gain.

Nevertheless, a nagging question remains. A major source of payment for the additional services were the Foundation grant and the Medicare and Medicaid waivers. Query: Once these funds run out, as they will in the near future, what are the implications of a marketing effort that stimulated demand which may not be sustained at the end of the demonstration? The question is easier raised than answered. One possible response is that if the additional services were needed—and many indubitably were—then it was justified to provide them, with the expectation that new and different dollars would replace the demonstration funds. That, however, raises a related question: Whether and to what extent the increased utilization of the centers was at the expense of other providers, public or private, individual or institutional, and thus did not necessarily provide significant net additional benefits.

A major source of strength for the demonstration was the inherent flexibility in its design which enabled each of the cities to develop a proposal following the model that best suited its environment and permitted modifications as the demonstration got under way. As our baseline study, *Urban Health Care for the Urban Poor* (1983), revealed, the participating cities varied with respect to the managerial and operating structures they had elaborated for the provision of ambulatory care to the indigent during the earlier decades when they had the support of federal and local targeted funds. In recognition of these differences, MHSP did not impose any singular model, but permitted each of the participating cities to develop a proposal for meeting the objectives of the program following a model suited to its needs and environment. Similarly, the grantees had considerable scope for adapting the initial proposal to the dictates of their experience during its implementation.

The variability in provider arrangements was substantial. In Cincinnati, the city had long had an extensive network of preventive and maternal and child care clinics under the aegis of its health department, some operated directly by the city, others by community-based groups. Several of the sites were selected to participate in the MHSP, whose chief programmatic objective was the establishment of a system-wide computerized billing and patient information system that was expected to improve quality control and efficiency. San Jose offered a sharp contrast in its choice of participants. There independent community groups were the sponsors of a number of neighborhood clinics and their satellites that were designated as recipients of the Foundation's support. In Baltimore, Milwaukee, and St. Louis, the focus of the program was upon modification of relations within the local government and the private sector to establish and expand the clinics that were included within the MHSP.

The functionalism of this high degree of local autonomy in developing the original model and in modifying it in the course of the demonstration was nowhere better demonstrated than when a period of crisis overtook the program. Two cities encountered serious financial problems, one involving arrangements with an outside major contractor engaged in capital improvement, the other arising from deviant accounting practices followed by one of the participating centers which ultimately was dropped from the program. In another city, radical and uncoordinated action by the community went a fair distance to undermining the program but the city was able to contain some of the ensuing turmoil and to make compensatory arrangements that sustained the program. Still elsewhere, the program was able to survive—even to expand—despite a prolonged political conflict focussed on the city hospital which paralyzed the municipal budget and subsequently toppled the mayor. In retrospect, it is certain that the flexibility built into the original design was a major asset in launching the program and in protecting it during crises that required difficult decisions and organizational reform.

The final issue that this evaluation will consider relates to the origins of the demonstration and its implications for the future. The Robert Wood Johnson Foundation adopted as its basic program orientation in the early 1970s the improvement of access to the health care system with a special focus on primary care. Its decision in the mid-1970s to explore the feasibility of an effort that evolved into the MHSP was consonant with the overall interests of the Foundation. But it would be an error to ignore the dilemma that the Foundation faced in making this decision and to overlook the measures that it took to strengthen the odds for the success of the demonstration.

What were the particular constraints inherent in the Foundation's decision to invest funds in the improvement of ambulatory care for inner-city populations? In the first place, there was no way that it could pursue its objective directly and independently. The medical infrastructure in most inner cities was sparse, deteriorating, or fragile. Further, city and county governments that were legally responsible for care of their indigent citizens furnished services that were limited both quantitatively and qualitatively. Many of the residents in the inner-city were recent immigrants, the majority of them members of groups with little economic and less political power. City and county governments had, since the years of the Great Society, depended upon the federal government for funds and other resources to improve health services to the indigent but by the mid-1970s the flow from Washington had begun to dry up.

Many of the public health facilities, particularly city and county hospitals, were seriously deteriorated and lacked both up-to-date equipment and competent staff. As a result of the freedom of provider choice offered to beneficiaries of the Medicare and Medicaid programs, the massive infusion of additional health dollars had not effected any substantial strengthening of the urban health infrastructure, in fact it may have undermined many preexisting resources.

Confronted with so many negative factors in the local environment, perhaps the most important judgment that can be made about the program is that the Foundation was willing to move ahead.

The second important observation is the skill and sophistication with which it moved. Had it not elicited the cosponsorship of both the U.S. Conference of Mayors and the American Medical Association, it is uncertain that the program would have gotten off the launching pad. A still more important step was negotiating the collaboration of the HCFA whose direct financial contribution to the demonstration via the Medicare waivers exceeded the Foundation's. By authorizing the Medicaid waivers HCFA encouraged the states as well to add several million dollars beyond their normal reimbursement to the centers. All of these were essential inputs.

Moreover, the Foundation, in accordance with its established practice, provided for a comprehensive evaluation of the program, to be performed by two university research teams; one concentrating on the political and institutional dimensions, the second on utilization and costs. Lacking sound systematic evaluation, the program could have little influence upon urban health care policy beyond the immediate confines of the participating sites.

The substantive question, then, is whether what we have learned from this five-year, five-city demonstration provides a sound basis for advocating concentration of the nation's efforts to improve the quantity and quality of health care services for the urban poor on strengthened neighborhood-based primary care centers. And if the answer is in the affirmative, what concomitant adjustments should be made in the extant delivery system and how can they be accomplished? This will be the subject of the next—and concluding—chapter.

7

The Potential of the Community Health Center

Our assessment of the Municipal Health Services Program, the five-year demonstration designed and funded by the Robert Wood Johnson Foundation with the aim of strengthening primary care delivery to inner-city populations, does not provide unequivocal findings that point to a singular policy direction. It would, in fact, have been surprising had the outcome been clear-cut and definitive in light of the variability among the five demonstration sites with respect to such key factors as size of the population in need, preexisting health resources, political leadership, and financial capability.

There is a second reason for the inability of the assessment to yield conclusive policy directions. During the five-year period of the demonstration and the years immediately following, the health care environment has been undergoing radical transformation. To note just a few major new developments:

- The moderating demand for health care services at a time when increasing numbers of physicians are entering practice and the nation's hospitals must contend with a large number of vacant beds.
- Advances in medical knowledge and technology, reinforced by cost pressures, that are resulting in the shift of a large volume of treatment to ambulatory settings and a further reduction in the demand for inpatient care.
- The shift in the political climate at both federal and state levels which has led to tax ceilings and tax reductions and thus diminished the funding available for social welfare programs, including appropriations for Medicaid.

- The development of new forms of health care delivery, in particular prepayment plans, aimed at providing acceptable care at an affordable price.

The challenge that this chapter faces is to relate the major findings from the experience of the five demonstration projects to the changing health care environment in order to formulate the preferred directions for public policy that will assure that health services to the urban poor are maintained and, in fact, improved.

As a point of departure, it may be useful to note those findings that are critical to the search for a strengthened system of care for the poor.

- The number and proportion of the inner-city population having no regular access to health care services turned out to be considerably smaller than was originally assumed.
- The number of active private practitioners in or adjacent to low-income areas was greater than had been anticipated and many of the poor and the near-poor could rely on them for some or all of their medical care.
- Many of the inner-city poor had long sought medical care from the emergency room or clinics of the municipal hospital although they lived outside its catchment area and continued to do so even after services became available at neighborhood health centers.
- Both the new and expanded community health centers were able over the years to increase their utilization to a level at which the calculated costs of the services they provided were considerably below the ambulatory care costs of the municipal hospital.
- The ability of the centers to provide both preventive and therapeutic services within the same setting was a boon to patients, particularly to mothers with young children and to the elderly.
- The financial viability of the centers depended in large measure on the Foundation subvention ($3 million per city over the five-year period) and the additional revenues generated by the Medicare and Medicaid waivers. The centers had relatively little success in attracting privately insured and self-pay patients.
- It was not feasible to shift resources from the municipal hospital to the centers with the increase in the patient load of the centers, as the project design had contemplated. What happened, instead, was an expansion in the total volume of ambulatory services to the poor and a concomitant reduction in the use of inpatient services by center enrollees.
- Since most of the funding for the centers derived from state, federal, and Foundation sources, the mayor proved to be a less powerful force for reform than had initially been conceived. In three of the five cities, control and operation of the public hospital were not within the jurisdiction of the municipality and this weakened the mayor's influence to restructure services and to reallocate resources.

Important as the foregoing findings are, they do no more than set the stage for the identification and assessment of alternative policies to provide acceptable, affordable care to the urban poor in the tumultuous years ahead during which the American health care system will be significantly altered.

We will begin by distinguishing between two sets of changes in the health care system, those that are more likely and those that are less likely to occur. Such an approach will serve to delineate the health care environment within which modifications must be sought in the decade ahead.

The following are some of the more probable changes:

- The nation's largest cities will experience a decline in the size of their inner-city populations, including the poor and the near-poor. The number of inner-city poor may stabilize or even decline in many cities with 500,000 to 1,500,000 inhabitants. Nevertheless, the one almost certain demographic conclusion is that there will continue to be considerable numbers of inner-city poor who have need for access to no-cost and low-cost health services.
- The nation's supply of physicians which amounted to 140 per 100,000 population in 1950 and is now nearing the 220 mark, will probably reach 260 by 1995 and may even go higher than that.
- The federal government which currently contributes more than half of the funds for Medicaid faces a steadily increasing budgetary stringency and this almost certainly assures efforts to constrain future outlays for health entitlement programs, both Medicaid and Medicare. As far as the states are concerned, if past be prologue, they too will aim to control their expenditures for health care since Medicaid has represented one of the fastest growing components of their budgets.
- The introduction of DRGs, the growth of for-profit medical enterprises, and the concerns of employers to constrain the costs of health care premiums are among the many new forces that are making the health care market more competitive and more price sensitive. Inner-city voluntary hospitals that traditionally provided a considerable amount of charity care, particularly ambulatory services, are under increasing pressure to cut back as they face a more competitive environment. They are forced to pay closer attention to their bottom lines.
- In response to mounting pressures from the purchasers of insurance to restrain their premium outlays, commercial insurance companies are moving aggressively to reduce the practice of "cross subsidization" which has enabled many voluntary hospitals to cover part of the cost of unrequited services to the poor.
- In the face of a damping demand for health care and increasing numbers of physicians and excess beds, many providers are exploring new delivery systems that aim to "lock in" a steady flow of insured patients. Even Medicaid patients present a potentially attractive market to many providers.

So much for the trends that are most likely to be strengthened in the decade ahead. We will now turn to others that may emerge but whose impact on the health care environment is uncertain.

- To start once again with demographics: A large stream of immigrants, legal and illegal, enter the United States each year; most of them locate in urban centers; and most of them are poor and will remain poor during their initial years here. What is more, many present or develop health problems that, if neglected, are a danger to themselves and also to others in their environment. Illegal immigrants threatened with apprehension and deportation, avoid, except in an emergency, seeking care in government facilities. It is not clear whether Congress which attempted to revise our immigration statutes in 1984 and failed, will try soon again; if so, whether it will succeed; and, if passed, what success such legislation will have in moderating the continuing large-scale inflow.

- The future rate of economic growth, the major determinant of the demand for labor, will have a significant impact on the rate of immigration, on individual and family incomes, and on the tax revenues of the different levels of government. Optimists are sanguine about our expanding economy but the trend data strongly suggest that the country will face another recession before the end of the 1980s. If there should be a loss of confidence in the dollar among foreign investors and the debts of the underdeveloped countries are not restructured, our economy may be seriously derailed. And should an economic slowdown persist for a number of years, the problems of providing adequate health care for the urban poor will be greatly compounded.

- There is broad agreement in the Congress that with the presidential election decided, it must soon address the unfavorable outlook for the Medicare Trust Fund. The Reagan administration is on record as favoring much larger user-payments by hospitalized patients and Congress, when it acts, is likely to reduce current benefits at the same time that it votes new earmarked taxes. It is not clear yet what combination of benefit reductions and new taxes Congress will adopt but it is reasonable to assume that the elderly will be required to pay more out of pocket for their health care.

- Numerous demonstrations are under way in different parts of the country aimed at enrolling both Medicaid and Medicare beneficiaries in prepayment plans, with the expectation of controlling costs and at the same time providing patients with more appropriate care. It is too early to assess the potential of these approaches. We know, however, that a prepayment plan is unlikely to succeed unless it can be protected from adverse selection. And the failure of the Commonwealth Health Care Corporation, Boston's well-designed prepaid health care program for Medicaid beneficiaries, has shown us the high value that many low-income persons place on retaining their freedom of choice in the selection of providers. Nevertheless, several states have moved to limit provider options for Medicaid enrollees and others are likely to follow.

- Some states, such as New York, Massachusetts, and Florida, have established all-payer systems designed to create a pool of revenue dollars which is redistributed among the member providers in proportion to their charity cases and bad debts. While this approach is still too recent for a balanced assessment, it offers the prospect of enabling voluntary hospitals with a long commitment to the urban poor to continue to serve them without running the risk of insolvency.

- There is a slow but steady movement toward withdrawal of local government from active hospital operation by selling out to a for-profit chain or occasionally, as in Baltimore, transferring the municipal hospital to a nonprofit sponsor. Such actions have been more frequent in smaller-sized communities but there have been instances where city or county government in a large metropolitan area has ceased to provide hospital care. As between political pressures to keep public hospitals operating and budgetary pressures to relieve local government of the burden of escalating hospital expenditures, it is difficult to outguess what the future balance will be.

Having delineated the probable and the uncertain trends in the future health care environment, we are now better prepared to address the central policy question: What would be the preferred way for urban communities to provide an acceptable level of ambulatory care to their inner-city poor in the decade ahead? More specifically, what should be the role of community health care centers in the evolving urban health care system?

Although it was a major programmatic initiative of the Great Society, the effort to establish a nationwide network of community health care centers never realized its ambitious goal of becoming the preferred provider of ambulatory care to inner-city populations. What is more, even after Medicare and Medicaid reimbursement became available to many inner-city inhabitants, few of these centers were able to achieve and maintain financial independence. Almost all must rely, to a greater or lesser degree, on annual subsidies. At the same time, it is evident that many community health centers provide a desirable level of care in convenient locations to inner-city families and have been able to build up and retain a satisfied patient clientele—a fact that is supported by the experience of the five-city MHSP demonstration. The first question that must be answered is whether in a period of continuing, probably increasing, financial stringency, existing centers should continue to be subsidized and new funds invested in establishing others. There is no one answer that would be appropriate given the diversity of the centers that are currently operating in different cities.

Part of the answer must be pragmatic. If a community has high regard for its health care centers, if large numbers of neighborhood residents are satisfied with the services that they receive, and if government and/or philanthropy can be persuaded to meet their annual deficits, there is good reason for the centers to continue operating.

A more complicated policy question arises if the existing level of funding for both the municipal hospital and the community health centers is cut back, and total inpatient and ambulatory care capacity must be reduced. Current trends in medical practice and in economics suggest that a reduction in the number of inpatient beds would be the preferred first order accommodation. The second order response would be to identify those ambulatory care facilities that could most readily be contracted or eliminated, based on location and user preferences. The experience of the MHSP has indicated that, other things being equal, the cost of ambulatory care in the neighborhood centers is considerably less than that of emergency room and outpatient care at the public hospital. But things are often not equal. Centers are unable to provide emergency care for trauma and to treat ambulatory patients with complicated diseases. As long as it remains necessary and desirable to operate the municipal hospital as a provider of last resort for the poor, the preferred choice may be to close one or more centers, especially if they have low levels of utilization and require substantial subsidies.

The recommendation that logic justifies the continued support of effectively functioning community health care centers does not imply support for their expansion. In a decade which will see a rapidly increasing supply of physicians, it is possible, even likely, that some new entrants into the profession will explore, in association with colleagues, the feasibility of establishing a group practice in or close to an inner-city neighborhood. Since such independent practice arrangements can provide ambulatory care services to patients at an average visit cost considerably below that of most community health centers, they should be favored over a program of center expansion. This conclusion, however, does not preclude support for the establishment of a new center in a neighborhood with no ready access to ambulatory care and where physicians, either individually or as members of a group, are unwilling to locate. In the absence of practitioners and with no hospital in the neighborhood, the establishment of a new center, particularly if it has substantial community approval, may offer the best opportunity to improve access to health care services for the local population.

All levels of government, particularly state governments, are following intently demonstrations aimed at enrolling Medicaid patients in prepaid delivery systems either by choice or by compulsion. Since the development, growth, and fiscal integrity of prepaid plans are always difficult to achieve, particularly if their enrollment is limited to or contains a high percentage of Medicaid patients, these plans must usually be founded on an existing institutional base, either a public or voluntary hospital, a community health center, or some similar agency. Even if government is willing to assume some of the development costs during the interval when the plan is building its enrollment and will also provide other types of assistance, the difficulties of launching a successful prepayment plan should not be minimized. In the final phase of the MHSP, when the demonstration was drawing to an end, there were scattered instances of physician groups who were exploring the feasibility of reorganizing into a capitated delivery system that would provide coverage for both Medicare and Medicaid beneficiaries whom they had been treating in the local center. Despite the substantial difficulties of moving in this direction, such efforts should not be written off.

Another development on the horizon is the perceived need of selected voluntary hospitals that face a declining inpatient census to assure themselves of a pool of prospective referrals. Accordingly, some are devising programs for the delivery of ambulatory care services at satellite locations, including community health centers, with the expectation that these will enable the hospital to maximize its inpatient load.

The foregoing are suggestive of the new departures in the provision of ambulatory care, currently in demonstration form if not in full-blown operation, that involve viable delivery modes for the inner-city. Each year is likely to see further innovations, now that patients with coverage are becoming an economic asset to the swollen ranks of physicians, to hospitals facing declining censuses, and to governments that are attempting to slow, or preferably from their vantage, to cap their health care outlays. In this environment, there is a continuing place for established community health centers that are operating close to the break-even point and the conditions exist that would justify new centers despite the strong desire of government to avoid new outlays for health care.

The thrust of the foregoing policy analysis, however, has been to call attention to alternative sources of health care delivery in the inner-city that hold substantial promise. To begin with, we have noted that the population in many inner-cities is more likely to remain stable or to decline than to increase. In light of the finding of the MHSP that as long as five years ago few inner-city residents were without access to health care, the only reasonable conclusion is that future demand will increase little, if at all, and it may even decline. In such an environment there is no clear need for the establishment of new centers. However, there is always room to provide more and better services for longer hours of the day and more days in the week. Another unequivocal finding from the MHSP experience was the ability of the centers to expand their patient load rapidly with the introduction of new services, preventive and therapeutic, as the result of the Foundation grant and the Medicare and Medicaid waivers.

There is no evidence as of early 1985 that either the federal government or state governments contemplate the perpetuation of these waivers for the centers that participated in the MHSP and surely no indication that they might extend them to others. Therefore, the centers are more likely to face a cutback than an expansion in the range of the services that they will be able to offer. It may turn out that centers that have enrolled a substantial number of Medicare patients and others with incomes above poverty level will be able to continue to offer some of the additional waivered services on a fee-for-service basis or through a prepayment arrangement.

Unless the American economy experiences vigorous growth for the next five to ten years that is reflected in a strong demand for labor, sizable gains in personal income, and enlarged government revenues—an unlikely but not impossible scenario—it is reasonable to expect some shrinkage in the number of existing centers and a reduction in the range of services that they provide. Only an occasional new center is likely to be established.

The preceding analyses and recommendations have focussed primarily on inner-city health centers that treat Medicare and Medicaid patients. We know, however, from the MHSP and from other sources that many people who use these centers are uninsured and are able to pay only part of their charges and not infrequently, nothing. We also know from the MHSP experience that the centers failed to attract significant numbers of non-Medicare and non-Medicaid patients with broad insurance coverage that would have enabled them to set their charges above costs and use the excess revenue to help defray the costs of care for the uninsured.

One of the chief reasons that even long-established and well-run community health centers have been dependent—some more, some less—on subsidies, has been their inability to cover with their operating revenues the free or below-cost care that they provide for the uninsured. Our society is now confronted with the need to explore the alternatives that exist, or might be put into place, to assure that all of the inner-city poor, including persons who are not eligible for Medicaid, can secure the basic health care services that they require.

Since the passage of Medicaid in 1965, the care of the uninsured poor has been met differently in different cities—by municipal or county hospital(s), voluntary hospitals located in low-income neighborhoods that have a tradition of serving the poor, community health centers usually assisted by government and philanthropic subsidies, or by other freestanding or satellite clinics. As voluntary hospitals have come under increasing financial pressure, the proportion of free care that they have been able to provide has declined, shifting more of the responsibility for charity care to the public hospitals and subsidized community health centers. In order not to reduce the number of providers willing to treat the uninsured poor, several states have in recent years moved, with the help of waivers from HHS, to establish all-payer systems which provide at least partial reimbursement to institutions that perform substantial amounts of charity care. Prior to the implementation of this cooperative financing mechanism, New York and some other states had allocated special funds for the same purpose; the program was known as "Ghetto Medicine."

Other attempts are underway to explore the potential of "insuring" the uninsured with the help of state and/or private funding, the latter usually contributed jointly by insurance providers following some distributive formula. But as various analyses have made clear, the difficulties are formidable in developing designs that do not lead to dysfunctional outcomes.

The final alternative is one that in recent years has virtually disappeared from the nation's health agenda, but it may yet return; that is, one or another form of national health insurance which would provide some level of coverage for the entire population. In the event that universal coverage were available and the principle of freedom of choice that currently prevails in most of the health care system were preserved, community health centers would probably be strengthened and their future secured through their ability to receive reimbursement for the treatment of all their patients, including those currently unable to pay. It would be a mistake, however, to assume that this would be the sole outcome of universal insurance. Such a radical political and economic transformation would likely lead to a great many other changes in the health care system that might either strengthen or weaken the role of community health care centers.

A note from history: In extended discussions with Aneurin Bevan, the father of Great Britain's National Health Service in the late 1940s, I challenged the enthusiasm for community health centers by suggesting that in a capital-tight system, the funds needed to build a network of such facilities might not be available immediately, if ever. It was more than a quarter of a century before Britain was able to establish even a few centers.

We can now sum up our principal recommendations on the future role of community health centers and our assessment of their performance potential in the changing health care environment.

- Since the early 1960s a large number of community health centers have been established and many of them have contributed substantially to providing improved ambulatory care for low-income inner-city populations. Even the most efficiently operated centers have, almost without exception, been dependent on annual subsidies to help them balance their books, partly because of the considerable volume of charity care that they provide to the uninsured. In the case of a center which provides a significant volume of ambulatory care to a user population that is satisfied with the services they receive, and which requires an annual subsidy that is not an excessive burden to the government and/or philanthropic funders, the preferred policy should be to assure its continuing operation. It would be desirable that the center explore new relationships with physician groups practicing in the neighborhood, with other centers, and with nearby hospitals, both public and voluntary, in order to improve referral systems and follow-up arrangements that would result in more and better care at lower total cost.

- In light of the stable or declining populations in most inner-city areas, the increasing pressures for fiscal constraint, and the growing numbers of physicians, a policy of restraint should be followed towards the establishment of new centers. This recommendation should not be read as blanket opposition to any additions, but rather as cautionary advice. With a large number of young physicians seeking opportunities for practice, with considerable momentum in the direction of prepaid delivery systems, and with other innovative approaches to health care delivery, the prospects are good that these alternatives may be able to provide more and better services at a lower unit and annual cost per patient.

- It is important in a period of cost constraint that the public hospital with its emergency room and specialty clinics remain as provider of last resort for the urban poor. Valuable as effective community health centers are, they cannot substitute for the broader services of the public hospital and its ambulatory clinics. Hence the future of the community health center must be assessed not only on its performance as an independent health care modality, but also on its role within the totality of the health care system available to the urban poor. Health care delivery for the poor is the function, in the first instance, of the public health care system, but it also involves other providers—from private physicians to voluntary hospitals.

- Finally, it is important that private third-party payers and the local philanthropic leadership explore and support all-payer systems which offer the best opportunity at this time and probably for the decade ahead, for all providers—public, nonprofit, and private—to cooperate in the care of the poor and particularly the uninsured. If the costs of charity care are not shared, an excessive burden will fall on the public sector; in a period of the cost constraint this would inevitably lead to serious deterioration in the quantity and quality of care available to the urban poor.

Community health centers have contributed to improved ambulatory care for the urban poor and with strong leadership they have the potential to make further advances. But in the rapidly changing urban and medical care environments that we have outlined, the community health center represents only one of a number of alternative providers and it should not be viewed as the sole or even the principal instrument for improving health care in the inner-city.

Index